THE HALF
DIET
DIET

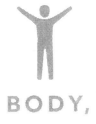 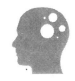

BODY, **MIND, AND SPIRIT**

FAMILIUS

Published by Familius LLC, www.familius.com

Familius books are available at special discounts for bulk purchases for sales promotions or for family or corporate use. Special editions, including personalized covers, excerpts of existing books, or books with corporate logos, can be created in large quantities for special needs. For more information, contact Premium Sales at 559-876-2170 or email specialmarkets@familius.com.

Library of Congress Cataloging-in-Publication Data
2015952350

Print ISBN 9781942934134
Ebook ISBN 9781942934622
Hardcover ISBN 9781942934639

Printed in the United States of America

Edited by Lindsay Sandberg
Cover design by David Miles
Book design by Brooke Jorden

10 9 8 7 6 5 4 3 2 1

First Edition

RICHARD EYRE

WITH FOREWORD BY DR. NOALL WOLFF

THE HALF DIET DIET

THE GUARANTEED WEIGHT-LOSS PROGRAM THAT REBOOTS YOUR

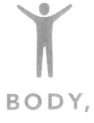

BODY, MIND, AND SPIRIT

GUARANTEE TO ALL READERS AND IMPLEMENTERS:

1. You will lose weight—quite a lot of weight in most cases.

2. Your weight loss will actually be the least important thing this book does for you.

3. If 1 and 2 don't prove to be true, I will personally give you your money back.

AUTHOR'S NOTE

This book was originally written online in weekly installments under the pen name of "Dr. Bridell." One advantage of writing a book bit by bit and putting each of its parts instantly online is that you get abundant, real-time feedback. I received thousands of comments, insights, and preorders for the first edition of the book. And I also received documented results of the weight being lost and other impressive results of the Half Diet.

Here, as "appetizers," are a few of those comments and testimonials, with names shortened to initials for privacy. There are many more at the end of the book for "dessert." You don't need to "eat" them all; just sample a few to get a taste of the nature and practicality of *The Half-Diet Diet*.

Bon appétit!

PRAISE FOR
THE HALF-DIET DIET

"Dear Dr. Bridell, I know you get lots of letters of gratitude for helping people lose weight. I want to thank you for something else. Thanks for teaching me how to enjoy food. Eating is now a delight, even though (or perhaps because) I eat only half as much as I used to. And guess what? You are right about food being a metaphor, because in learning how to enjoy eating, I have learned how to enjoy life!" —RM

"A life-changing approach to weight loss." —MS

"I love the insights about the spiritual aspects of our relationship to food." —LJ

"I know this 'diet' works! It's totally in harmony with the spiritual truth. So how can it not work?!" —JH

"I've truly enjoyed your columns and especially appreciate how the three parts dovetail (the physical, mental, and spiritual). I didn't need to lose weight, but the slowing down and appreciating all aspects of my life have helped me be 'more at peace' with myself." —LH

"I found hope on both the physical and spiritual level. I am so grateful for this book. It has given me the only hope I have felt in years of dieting." —FB

"I loved it all, but especially the second half of the book . . . on the spiritual appetites." —FG

"It is definitely more than a food issue for me. I like the spiritual approach to focus on life management." —LM

"Deeply insightful and thought provoking." —HD

"From the beginning, I have felt that this is the answer for me because I had come to the realization that my weight issue and my spiritual progress are tied together." —MM

"It has been so refreshing to see a common-sense and reasonable way to handle weight problems. I am grateful as one of those who are fed up with the usual 'diet' fads and have appreciated your wonderful ideas. They have worked miracles in my life." —CW

"I began reading it because I was interested in losing weight, but my motivation became much deeper as the weeks went by." —DC

"Enlightening, thought-provoking, and enjoyable." —SB

"As a physician, I say thanks for your work and insight. I agree with your concepts and fundamental ideas." —LS

"It's the first diet that has articulated what I have always believed a diet should be. Yes, it works, because it encompasses the total person and not just the physical side of dieting." —BN

"I especially appreciate the fact that you are using spiritual principles and examples to help us understand our behavior, desires, motivations, etc. Not only does it help people eat better and lose weight, but, hopefully, [it] also improve[s] their spirituality and strength to endure." —CH

Endorsements continued in back of book . . .

MEDICAL FOREWORD

First of all, you should know that my friendship with Richard Eyre goes back forty years. He calls me "Cub," and I call him "Rick." We ride horses together, we scuba dive together, and, mostly, we talk a lot together, particularly about the maintenance and the connections of the bodies, minds, and spirits we are trying to preserve. You should also know that I love the way Rick's logical and conceptual mind works. His how-to advice has been a constant source of practical information to me throughout my life, but even more, it's frequently given me a sense of "Ah-ha!" joy.

About me: I'm nothing more than an average country doctor. Way back in the last century, I started my medical practice in a little country town in Alberta, Canada. I could immediately see that obesity was a universal problem and a bane to most of my patients. A friend of mine from medical school had a diametrically opposite experience. He went directly to Nigeria with his new wife and stayed there for sixteen years as a medical missionary. He was one of two doctors that spoke the language of the Tieve, a tribe of a million and a half people in which obesity is nonexistent.

On one of his rare trips back home, we got together and discussed the differences in our medical experiences. I found that for him there were no Sundays and no holidays and that on a typical day he and his partner would see five hundred outpatients. Now when I say "outpatient," I mean *out*. There is no possible way to funnel that many patients through a typical doctor's office. These patients would literally stand in an almost endless line, and my friend would run down the line giving instructions to his Nigerian nurses. "You know what to do with this one, this one is routine. Oh! This one needs immediate surgery; take her to the OR—she needs a cesarean section immediately." During his stay in Nigeria, his surgical schedule would include seven or eight major cases each day. Obviously, this kind of crushing schedule can only be maintained by an individual with unusual physical stamina. During all these years, he and his family lived on a typical Nigerian diet: millet, yams, and a chicken every couple of weeks.

Now imagine the kind of woman who could be the wife to such a doctor: bearing and raising children and sticking with that man and being his active partner. That couple, the doctor and his wife, not only had unusual physical stamina but also a deep well of spiritual, social, and intellectual durability. They would have loved Rick's "diet book" because it raises the bar of all the diet books that have previously been written—it includes advice not only on how to live but on how to serve with heart, might, mind, and strength.

My friend says that he thinks he may have seen a heart attack once in his sixteen years in the Nigerian village. Imagine a typical American doctor who had only seen one heart attack in sixteen years! Try to imagine that American or Western doctor never having seen a case of adult onset diabetes. Imagine that doctor having "seen hemorrhoids only in a book." Imagine a scenario where cancer of the colon is almost unknown.

As we compared notes, my friend from Nigeria and I realized he was spending most of his time treating diseases that had been eradicated in the West. He averaged one cesarean section a day because of rickets. I have not seen as much vitamin D deficiency in my fifty-year medical career as he saw in one day. We came to the conclusion that I was treating "civilized diseases" that he never encountered in Nigeria—arteriosclerosis, type 2 diabetes, cancers of the bowels, fibromyalgia, chronic pain syndromes, osteoporosis, and so on. Every one of the diseases I constantly treated (and he never treated) were related, in large part, to diet.

In my own early practice, I became something of a "bariatric specialist" before the specialty was invented. This was because I realized that if I could just get my ubiquitously overweight patient population on a good diet, I could prevent most of the diseases I was treating. I knew how the chemistry worked; I had a minor in biochemistry and knew every step of the tricarboxylic acid cycle with its associated enzymes, coenzymes, and sidechains allowing the metabolism of protein and fat, all for the production of high-energy phosphate bonds needed for muscular contraction.

So as a young doctor, I educated myself on every diet available. I studied the diets celebrities use, the South Beach diet, the Atkins high-protein modified fast, hypnosis and self-hypnosis, pins in the earlobe which you pull when you're hungry, daily shots of human chorionic gonadotropin and a 400-calorie diet, etc., etc., etc. Over the years, I have caused tons of weight to be lost. And over all those years, I have come to realize that permanent weight loss will require not only dietary changes but fundamental changes in brain chemistry. You must literally become a thin person in the mind. You must learn how to charge the reticular activating system with mild exercise, how to change the pleasure centers in the brain from the cortisol whirlpool to the endorphin cascade. A whole new mindset will require the same gradual changes in brain chemistry and brain morphology that occur in a recovering alcoholic.

Rick has captured this new mindset, and he has done so in a clear and simple way that would have been impossible for me with my medical terminology and scientific baggage!

In the past, I've told my patients not to try making changes in behavior until they were really ready to make those changes. This is exactly the wrong advice. Change now, change today, change this instant, make plans to use the tools you have right now, and if you fail, start again and again and again. Ask questions, learn from your mistakes, and start again. The more often you try to change, the more certain you can be that, eventually, you will. And it is this very book that will make it all possible.

Years ago, when Rick told me that he was tired of "fad diets," I agreed with him. When he told me he was about ready to write a diet book of his own, I encouraged him. And when he told me he wasn't sure he had the medical or dietary credentials, I said, "Rick, your freedom from the narrowed perspective of ever-changing nutritional and medical science is the very reason you should write the book."

Frankly, we've got too many scientists and pseudoscientists pumping out incomplete and illogical dieting theories that ignore things like the joy of eating and the need for balance and moderation and simple common sense.

What this world needs is a straightforward program for turning our appetites into our friends rather than our enemies and for exercising simple discipline—not to curtail but to enhance our joy of the physical world, including the parts of it that we eat!

A true and useful lifetime diet must involve the health of the mind and spirit as well as the body and must increase the joy we get from eating, not diminish it.

And that is exactly what the Half Diet does!

Based on correct principles rather than passing theories, this diet not only legitimately guarantees weight loss, but also promises more energy, higher awareness levels, and a carry-over talent for controlling all the other appetites that threaten our happiness.

One thing I've learned over the course of my fifty years of practicing medicine is that patients will not keep doing things that they don't enjoy and that don't make sense to them. The promises some diets make will hook people for a while, and some immediate results will keep them going a little longer, but without understanding why they are doing what they do, and without any noticeable improvement in how they feel emotionally as well as physically, they won't stick with it, and their weight will go up and down like a yo-yo as they flit from one diet fad to another.

The Half Diet is the antithesis of all that. It will work, *and* you will enjoy your food more and enjoy your life more.

I was honored to be asked to write the preface to this book, because I endorse and believe all that Richard has said herein. In fact, I like to think that I have contributed somewhat to it.

The most unique thing about the dietary approach that Rick suggests is that it works *with* the body and with the natural appetite rather than *against* them. It suggests that appetite is, like a strong and beautiful horse, something that can work to our benefit and to the enhanced pleasure of life if it is controlled or "bridled."

During all the years of my medical practice, I have tried to simplify the ideas of what to eat and what not to eat so that my patients could remember and implement rather than become discouraged and intimidated. The simplification went as far as "green food is good, eat it in abundance; brown food is okay, eat it moderately; white food is bad, try not to eat it at all." But Rick, in this book, has created an even more useful simplification. "Worry only about disciplining the quantity of what you eat, and over time your appetite will become your ally and attract you to a higher quality of food."

I agree with and endorse this concept: I agree that it is both simpler and more effective to focus on controlling *how much* you eat than on complex combinations and fastidious formulas for exactly *what* you should eat.

Hold in check the quantity, and your appetite will gradually stop demanding more and start demanding better. And the bonus is that while you are cutting in half the amount of food you eat, you will, counterintuitively, double the enjoyment you get in eating that half!

The problem, of course, is the transition. Your appetite will fight you—hard—when you start giving it less. So the real value of this book is the tips and ideas it lays out for "holding to half." You will like the water habit and the move habit and the slow habit because they will make your job of quantity control easier.

This book, long before it was published for the general public, was serialized in an online publication and met with huge acclaim. Those who tried it, who made the commitment to develop and follow the habits it suggests, met with real success. They lost weight, and they felt better about their bodies and about themselves. And they experienced few, if any, negative side effects other than the slight edge of hunger that actually quickens the wits and raises the levels of awareness and perspective.

I'll make you a little promise here at the outset: if you have the faith and the discipline to implement the Half Diet, full force, for a full month, you will develop positive dietary habits that can last a lifetime.

Enjoy the process,

Noall E. Wolff, MD

PREFACE TO THE SECOND EDITION

In some ways, this is actually a third edition, because most of *The Half-Diet Diet* was initially published in installments in a periodical and written under the pseudonym of "Dr. Bridell." The series was wildly popular and led me to put it in book form as the first edition, which generated still more input and feedback.

The reason I used a pseudonym is that I wanted people to focus on the actual principles of the diet, not on the author. After all, I've been a successful author who writes about families, marriage, parenting, and work/family balance, and I didn't want people saying, "What does that guy know about nutrition and diet?"

Since then, however, as people have thanked Dr. Bridell for helping them lose weight and master various appetites, I have realized that this book is entirely consistent with my other books—it *is* a book about families and marriage and balance, because our physical health and our appetite control and how well we take care of our own bodies, minds, and spirits are powerfully influential on how good a parent and spouse we are.

So I was emboldened, over time, to agree to this second edition, this time under my own name. Part of my new confidence came from the spectacular results and feedback I received on the diet. People who implement these practices are not just losing weight; they are keeping it off, and they are actually enjoying food more than they ever have before. The premise of the diet—that if you discipline the quantity of your intake, your body will gradually shift to demanding better quality instead—is working for those who develop the self-mastery to truly eat half.

And the underlying metaphor of the book—of how the horse (appetite) is good, not bad, and needs to be trained and bridled rather than killed—is making sense to those who really think about it. (The original pen name "Bridell" came from the metaphor of controlling a horse with a bridle.)

BUT, not all the feedback I got was positive. Here are some recent comments from frustrated readers:

- "I'm so mad; I just can't lose as much as I want as fast as I want."
- "I can't do this the rest of my life."
- "I know my body—only cutting carbs works for me."
- "How long do I have to do this? I'm getting so tired of eating like a bird."

Comments like this make me realize that so many don't really understand the basic principles involved here . . . and they also make me realize that the word *diet* may be part of the problem. People are conditioned to think of a diet as something short term and painful—something we torture ourselves with for a period of time so that we can reach some goal and then go back to our old, enjoyable ways. It is viewed as a trade-off. "I love eating, but I hate being fat, so I will give up eating for a while until I'm not fat."

This kind of dieting, up and down, is like living life on a roller coaster and ultimately probably does our bodies more harm than good (and certainly frustrates us out of our minds).

So if "diet" implies something short term, and something painful, it is the wrong word for the Half-Diet lifestyle. The Half Diet is about joy—about increasing the pleasure of eating (riding) and training the appetite (horse) to work for us rather than against us.

When a horse is ridden well, with the correct use of the bridle, it becomes more and more joyful to ride. The joy is progressive: it gets better and better. Once the horse knows the feel of the bridle, it stops trying to work against it. And when well trained, when a bridle has been used long enough and effectively enough, we get to a point where we can give the horse its head, knowing that it will not hurt us, only thrill us!

> The Half Diet is about joy—about increasing the pleasure of eating (riding) and training the appetite (horse) to work for us rather than against us.

That is the principle of *The Half-Diet Diet*. Bridle your appetite by drinking a big glass of water before each meal and by eating only half at three meals a day. Once the appetite knows that that is all it is going to get, it stops trying to work against you and actually starts craving better, more nourishing food. Since its job is to get enough nutrients, and since it can't have more quantity, it starts wanting more quality. And when we get it well trained, we get to a point where we know our appetites will work for us rather than against us and we increase our joy in food and in life!

Now think about that for a moment. When appetites are in the unbridled mode, they work on quantity; they want to be in charge, to run away with us. We find ourselves eating fast and taking big bites; we gulp, gorge, and guzzle—the appetite is winning! We are getting filled up, but there is little joy in it.

Now put on the bridle. Eat slowly; take small bites; sip, savor, and smell. Feel the texture of the food; notice the aftertaste. Set the fork down between small bites, and enjoy. Make the bites half as big, and take one half as often; it will take you twice as long to eat half the amount of food, and your enjoyment level will be much higher.

> Think of the Half-Diet Diet not as a diet at all but as a way of maximizing the joy you can get from your bridled appetite and from your God-given body. The joy comes not from satisfying or being controlled by your appetite but from bridling it and working with it and training it.

Then put the horse in the barn until it's time for the next ride. Don't let it go running around on its own. Don't pick up everything edible you see and put it in your mouth. If you need a snack between your slow, enjoyable half meals, eat an apple or a carrot. (Horses like those, you know, and so will your appetite, once you get it trained.)

Think of the Half-Diet Diet not as a diet at all but as a way of maximizing the joy you can get from your bridled appetite and your God-given body. The joy comes not from satisfying or being controlled by your appetite but from bridling it and working with it and training it. There is joy in this kind of mastery, and there are results that are lasting and that keep getting better and better. There is joy in smelling, sipping, and savoring good food, and in eating it slowly and with small bites, and in staying with the eat-half bridle.

Enjoy, and be thin . . .

Richard Eyre (a.k.a. Dr. Bridell)

Park City, Utah, 2016

CONTENTS

CANDOR, APPETITES, GUARANTEES, REASONS, AND RESULTS

Completely candid honesty! That's one of the things that sets this diet apart from the rest. So let's start with this: I'm not a doctor. I'm not a dietitian either, or an exercise therapist or anything else that would give me even the remotest credential for writing a diet book. What I am is a practical person who is interested mostly in results. I'm also a writer who keeps noticing that diet books are always on the best-seller lists. (And most of them promise far more than they can deliver and never address the emotional and spiritual *causes* of our physical problems.) What I like about the subject of dieting is that it's *current*, it's *present*, and it's about our daily habits and routines, about what you're going to eat today and tonight. It can help you start trying something new right now.

I don't know a thing about calories or fat grams or metabolism or antioxidants or even proteins or carbohydrates. In a way, this ignorance is bliss. I don't get confused about why the experts keep changing their minds about what is really good or bad for you. But I do know—absolutely—a couple of important things:

1. I know a way anyone can lose weight, for sure, for real, and keep it off and be healthier than ever before . . . and actually enjoy the process.

2. I know that there is a direct, unbreakable connection between human happiness and the control of human appetites—and I don't just mean the appetite for food.

So, again, I have no credentials, nothing other than my absolute, outlandish claim that I know a simple diet that really works, for everyone, and that the same principles that make the diet work also apply to other appetites and thus make other things work better too—like *life*!

Just how sure am I about this? Well, my initial assurance was based on the fact that the diet worked for me and for the family and friends that tried it. Then, as mentioned, the diet was serialized in an online magazine and the testimonials that poured in increased my belief that it was simple enough to work for anyone with the discipline to implement it. Some of the testimonials that poured in are included in the preface material and there are additional ones at the back of the book. Actually, the total weight loss, just of those column-readers who took the trouble to write in and tell me about it, was over two tons!

WHO SHOULD READ THIS BOOK?

Whom is this book for? Well, first, it's for folks who've tried other diets that didn't work, or didn't work for very long, or who heard about other diets and knew, without even trying them, that they wouldn't work or that they couldn't stand them or couldn't do them. And it's for people who want to go beyond food progress toward gaining control of all appetites. This book is for people who want a higher, more intelligent, more spiritual approach and who want to understand and then to win the greatest of all personal battles: the one between one's spiritual soul and one's physical appetites.

There are way too many diet books out there, and most of them, in the long run, do more harm than good. Lots of diet books, lots of promises, lots of different slants on the science of nutrition. This one is different. It will present a series of concepts, starting with the deceptively simple, and build to a deeper understanding of what a diet really should be and why it should be thought of spiritually rather than physically.

Whom is this book for? Well, first, it's for folks who've tried other diets that didn't work, or didn't work for very long. And it's for people who want to go beyond food progress toward gaining control of all appetites.

LEVELS

Remember as you read (particularly the first few chapters) that all physical things are "types" or metaphors for the deeper reality of the spiritual. I think God could have devised any number of methods for refueling our physical machines. We could have plugged into trees or had some kind of built-in solar batteries, but he gave us the *food* method, with all of its nuance and variety and with the marvelous aspects of taste and appetite. He gave us this because it is a way of learning some things about mastery and about the relationship between body and spirit that apply to all aspects of life and of eternity, and that provide us with the tools we need to find and to create the mortal joy we were sent here to find.

(If that last paragraph didn't make full and completely coherent sense, don't worry. After all, this is just the introduction. I promise you that by the end of the book, you will be able to go back and read the paragraph and it will seem absolutely elementary—and absolutely true.)

Maybe you've had a discussion like the one I had on an airplane the other day, sitting by a scientist I had just met who was telling me that man was just an advanced animal—perhaps not even the most advanced (she really liked dolphins). I must have looked disagreeable, because she challenged me to name a really substantive "difference in kind" between animals and humans (she had already minimized the physical and mental differences as "differences in degree"). Judging her to be unreceptive to spiritually oriented ideas, I tried this one: humans and animals are polar opposites—180-degree opposites—in terms of their purpose and the manner in which they maximize their potential. My punch line was this: "Animals become all they can be by following their instincts and appetites. Humans become all they can be by mastering and controlling their instincts and appetites."

> "Animals become all they can be by following their instincts and appetites. Humans become all they can be by mastering and controlling their instincts and appetites."

I want you to think of this diet as an exercise or an experiment in reaching your full potential. The food is just part of the laboratory or the gymnasium we call mortality. And the diet works on many levels, the first of which is the physical.

Remember, as you begin to read the chapters, that what this book really is about . . . is *joy* and *love*. And the best definition I know of joy is the winning of the ongoing battle between spirit and flesh, between discipline (or discipleship) and appetites.

ACT I

THE PHYSICAL
HALF DIET

There are lots of good reasons to go on a diet: to feel better, to think better, to work better, to play better, to look better, to live longer. The bottom line is that we really are what we eat, so there is genuine merit in having some kind of strategy for what we put in our mouths (and what we don't).

CHAPTER 1

THE BASIC CONCEPT OF THE HALF-DIET DIET

There are so many good, natural, tasty, nourishing things on this earth to eat, and guess what: your body *wants* and *needs* some of most of them and most of some of them. Diets that eliminate all the carbs, or all the proteins, or even all the fats are taking away things your body needs as well as wants.

At its best, your appetite, far from being your enemy, can be the sensor that tells you what your body needs. (Your appetite probably isn't doing that for you right now, because you've messed it up a bit. But you can fix it so the things that sound, look, smell, or taste the best to you actually are the best for you.) So the basic beginning premise of this book is that our appetites are good, our senses are good, the earth is good, and natural food, in all its variety, is good.

The problem is that appetites don't know when to quit. They tell us what we want, but they don't

> So the basic beginning premise of this book is that our appetites are good, our senses are good, the earth is good, and natural food, in all its variety, is good.

tell us how much of it we need. There's no overload bell or back-up beeper.

So here's the basic principle of the Half-Diet Diet, right here in the first chapter of this book: eat what you want, but only eat half of it (half of your normal portion, half of what your appetite wants).

As simple as that sounds, it makes eminent sense. Here's why:

On average, Americans eat about twice as much as they need.[1] Since the quantity is too high, the quality goes down. (That's because the body can get the same amount of what it needs out of twice as much bad food as it can out of half as much good food.)

> When you deny your body's demands for more quantity, it will start demanding more quality instead. Vegetables and fruits will gradually look better, and junk foods and "fluff" foods will start to look worse.

So what could be simpler? Eat what you want, but only eat half of it, half of what you are accustomed to eating. Over time (a fairly short time, actually), your body will adjust and start being more selective in what it tells you it wants, since it is getting only half as much. When you deny your body's demands for more quantity, it will start demanding more quality instead. Vegetables and fruits will gradually look better, and junk foods and "fluff" foods will start to look worse.

One unique thing about the Half-Diet Diet is that it's actually easiest to implement when you're eating out. At restaurants, you order what you want and they bring you, on average, two portions—twice as much as you need. You eat half of it—half of each thing on the plate.

By the way, if your mother, in addition to telling you to clean your plate, told you that the children in Africa would starve if you didn't finish your food, then you may have a hard time throwing half of your meal away. So have it boxed or wrapped up and give it to a homeless person on your way home or to your teenager or your dog when you get home. As a last resort, eat it yourself later on—but for an upcoming meal, not for a midnight snack.

The principle is the same for eating in as for eating out. Just make half. (Be honest—you know what half is!) If you're not the "maker," just take half servings.

In theory, the Half-Diet Diet is almost absurdly simple. Eat three "half meals" a day. (And you can also get away with a couple of half snacks.) But nothing else, nothing in between. What's hard is quitting when half is gone. It's hard to shut down, to not fudge. It's hard, but it gets gradually easier. Your discipline increases as your body (and stomach) adjusts.

That's it. That's the core and the essence of the physical Diet. The next few chapters are just a bunch of practical (and, in some cases, very creative) suggestions and methods to make it easier, more interesting, and more fun to "eat half."

To be clear, the Half Diet is not telling you what to eat or asking you to count calories or vitamins. The goal of "eat half" is to retrain your appetite to want quality food. But if you are concerned that half of your normal portion really is too little, that you aren't getting the nutrition that you need, talk with your doctor or dietitian and decide on a portion size that is appropriate for you.

And stick to it.

WHAT YOUR BODY WILL DO FOR YOU

With a concept as simple as the challenge in Chapter 1 (just continuing your life as is but cutting each thing you eat in half and stopping when that first half is gone), you'd think there would now be some much more complicated follow-up chapter that outlines just what you can and can't eat and telling you how to count fat grams or calories or carbs and instructing you to buy herbs or supplements or organic food. In other words, if Chapter 1 is about the quantity (eating half), then Chapter 2 must be about the quality, right?

Yes and no. Yes, this second chapter is about quality and nutrition, but no, it doesn't require you to count anything or plan elaborate menus or buy specific kinds of food. In fact, it isn't about you doing anything for your body. *It's about what your body will do for you* as a reward for the effort you make to eat half as much.

> As you continue to cut your intake in half, you will essentially be training and developing a more selective appetite.

As your body gets used to less *quantity,* it will start demanding more *quality.* Vegetables and fruits and grains will become more appealing. As you continue to cut your intake in half, you will essentially be training and developing a more selective appetite. Remember that you are not trying to kill or eliminate your appetite; rather, you're conditioning it so it will give you more joy and better results.

The secret to this whole diet is this: your body knows what it needs. Every cell in your body knows what it requires to stay alive and to thrive. It is this paradigm that sets the Half-Diet Diet apart from every other diet you could try. It puts the ultimate authority and knowledge of nutrition on the only source that actually knows what you need: your body.

Every person's metabolism and nutritional needs are different. Some need more protein; others thrive on carbs. Traditional diets appeal to some but fail for others because they ignore differences and try to put everyone into the same strict diet box. The Half Diet approach harnesses the perfect knowledge of your own body, which, when bridled, will tell you just what you need.

> The Half Diet approach harnesses the perfect knowledge of your own body, which, when bridled, will tell you just what you need.

But your body doesn't wrest control from your appetites and obsessions and bad habits *unless you train it to.*

The body is an instinctive mechanism. Unlike the mind, which can choose and determine its own thoughts, the body—untrained and ungoverned—will take the path of least resistance. Thus, if you're eating twice as much as you need, and much of it is junk food or other unhealthy stuff, your body doesn't fight you, so long as there's enough food coming in to provide what your cells need.

Say your body needs "3n" of nutrients each day and it can extract that much from a "6v" volume of fairly bad food. Your instinctive body is OK with that, even though half the volume may be making you fat or tired or full of cholesterol. If the food you're eating gets even worse in quality (say it now takes 8v volume to get the 3n of nutrients), your body will push you to eat even more.

But what happens if the mind takes control by enforcing the "eat half" principle and limits the body to 3v volume of food per day? If it's all the same fairly bad food, the body will be getting only 1.5n, and the appetite will push you to eat more. But if the mind stays strong and holds the quantity line at 3v, the only recourse your cells have is to work on the quality. Gradually, you will start craving better, more nourishing, more wholesome food until your body can get its 3n of nutrients from a volume of 3v.

n = nutrients

v = volume of food

3n = 6v or 3n = 3v

Consequently, if you stay true to eating half as much, your body will gradually give you the gift of craving quality instead of quantity. Your tastes (as well as your taste) will change, your body will lose weight, and every one of your cells will be happier.

Can it really be that simple? Absolutely! But simple things are often incredibly hard. How in the world are you going to eat only half as much food? If you've tried it for even a day or two, you know how hard it is! How can you do it—not for just a meal or a day or a week but from now on? It is an extremely difficult proposition because any weakness in your conscious, choice-making mind will be exploited mercilessly by your instinctive body and your subconscious appetites.

And nobody else can do it for you. No one can make it easy or give you some magic pill. What I can do for you, what this book is written to do, is to motivate you by making the whole idea of "eat half" as appealing as possible by giving

Eating twice as slowly and half as much is, as you get used to it, more enjoyable than the way you eat now.

you some interesting, stimulating, and new ways to think about it and by helping you see that it's not only the results that will make you happy but the process, that eating twice as slowly and half as much is, as you get used to it, more enjoyable than the way you eat now.

The thing to work on first is the "slow" part. Make your bites smaller and chew them longer, so that eating half as much takes as long as eating the full amount used to. Think quality over quantity. Sip, savor, and smell instead of guzzling, gulping, and gorging. But wait—we're getting ahead of ourselves; in fact, that is the title of the next chapter. See you there.

CHAPTER 3

SIP, SAVOR, AND SMELL; DON'T GUZZLE, GULP, AND GORGE

Let's start this chapter by thinking for a minute about how most dogs eat. It's pretty ugly. It's a race. It's like they're worried that something or someone will get their food before they can gulp it down. Their eyes dart around. They are protecting their food and trying to eat it before anyone else can get it or take it away. Taste, for most animals, seems to exist only in the form of salivating, instant gratification as they gorge, or maybe a warning that something they're trying to eat may be rancid or toxic. They bolt things down too fast to really taste them.

Unfortunately, our own eating patterns aren't as different from dogs' as they should be. We "snarf" our food, eating by instinct and appetite rather than by taste. Humans ought to eat in a completely opposite way from how animals eat.

As we explored in Chapter 2, there is something starkly simple and perfectly proportionate about the Half-Diet Diet. Eat half as fast (or twice as slowly), and it will then take the same amount of time to eat our half portions as it used to take to eat the whole thing. And as you get used to eating twice as slowly and half as much, you will crave half as much and enjoy the food you do eat twice as much. (Isn't it nice how every one of those "halves" and "twices" works in your favor?)

Most people say they enjoy eating, but hardly anyone makes a conscious effort to really appreciate and taste their food every time they eat. The three Gs—guzzling, gulping, and gorging—seem to be much more common than the three Ss— smelling, sipping, and savoring.

EATING AS AN ART

Eating can be, and should be, one of the best things in life, one of the simplest pleasures. When it is thought of and pursued as a pleasure, it is done slowly and observantly and it can involve all five senses. Good food's color and design and preparation can be appreciated by our eyes, its aroma by our noses, its texture by our touch, and its remarkable taste by our tongues and different parts of our mouths. Even the through-the-bone sounds of food being thoughtfully chewed can be part of the sensual symphony.

As with anything else in life, the more we pay attention to the finer points of eating, the more pleasurable the consumption of food becomes and the better we become at enjoying it. We also become more discerning, more discriminating, and thus more selective about what we eat.

> Eating can be, and should be, one of the best things in life, one of the simplest pleasures. When it is thought of and pursued as a pleasure, it is done slowly and observantly and it can involve all five senses.

When eating is routine, or habitual, or compulsory, we hardly taste or enjoy the food. We just stoke ourselves like throwing coal in a furnace; we fuel up like pumping gas into a car.

Sometimes, even when we do taste and savor our food, it's only for the first bite or two. We enjoy that initial taste and then settle into the routine of eating. A little of this "diminishing return" is natural; the first run down the ski hill is always the most exhilarating. But we can train ourselves to enjoy the last bite of a meal almost as much as the first. Part of how we do this is taking only half as many bites or, better yet, making every bite only half as big.

BY THE NUMBERS

Say a normal or average eater (guzzle, gulp, and gorge) eats a meal in twenty big, hurried bites. The first bite tastes good and every subsequent bite a little less good, until most of the meal is just refueling or obeying the appetite. Now, say a skilled and artistic eater (sip, savor, and smell) eats half as much but takes the time to really enjoy each bite, perhaps splitting his ten bites into twenty smaller, more tasted amounts. His enjoyment of each subsequent bite diminishes more slowly, and he ends up with twice the total pleasure, though he ate only half of the food. Let's say the numbers below represent the enjoyment factor of each bite. (The left column is the twenty bites of the guzzling, gulping gorger; the right column is the twenty divided or half-size bites of the smelling, sipping savorer.) Remember that since each bite on the right is half as big, the total food consumed in that column is half of the consumption on the left, yet the total enjoyment is twice as much.

GGG		SSS	
Bite Number	Enjoyment Factor	Bite Number	Enjoyment Factor
1	10	1	10
2	9	2	10
3	8	3	9
4	7	4	9
5	6	5	9

GGG		SSS	
Bite Number	Enjoyment Factor	Bite Number	Enjoyment Factor
6	5	6	8
7	4	7	8
8	4	8	8
9	4	9	7
10	4	10	7
11	3	11	7
12	3	12	6
13	3	13	6
14	2	14	6
15	2	15	5
16	2	16	5
17	1	17	5
18	1	18	5
19	1	19	5
20	1	20	5
Total Enjoyment	75	Total Enjoyment	150

Learn to take a little space between bites, like a lift ride between ski runs. Set your fork down between bites. Pause for a minute to reflect on the last bite and to anticipate the next. Like Edward Abbey, who loved the desert because its stark simplicity allowed him to focus on the beauty of one single cactus flower[2], we need to separate and isolate each bite. Don't run your bites together into an over-rich profusion of gluttony. Space them like the sparse and appreciated single cactus flower.

Paying attention, tasting, sipping, smelling, and savoring not only make eating more enjoyable, but they also force us to slow down. They replace quantity with quality, decreasing the former and increasing the latter. Someone who focuses on the three Ss will be more aware of the joy of good food. He will also notice things like the slightly unpleasant, greasy feeling in the mouth or the processed, preservative aftertaste of food we should eat less of.

> Learn to take a little space between bites, like a lift ride between ski runs. Set your fork down between bites. Pause for a minute to reflect on the last bite and to anticipate the next.

The trade-offs of the "eat half" approach are pretty good! You eat only half as much food, but you double how long you chew and how much you savor. As quantity goes down, both the quality of the experience and (over time) the quality of the food go up. You trade 50 percent of all the things that hurt (bulk, calories, fat, and everything excessive that's in there) for 100 percent more of all the things that help (enjoyment, time, discernment, and superior nutrients).

LESS IS MORE

If you still have some doubts about these "halvings" and "doublings," try the popcorn experiment:

First, prepare or buy a bag of buttered, salted popcorn. As you eat it, pay attention to *how* you eat it. If you are like most people, your bites will get progressively bigger as your appetite takes over. Your first bites will be two or three kernels in the tips of your fingers, but by the end, you will be eating handfuls.

Second, on another day, get another bag of the same popcorn and eat normally again, only this time, eat just half and throw the other half away. It will take some willpower, because you will be stopping just when your appetite is peaking and your bites are growing.

Third, on a third day, get yet another identical bag of popcorn, but this time, eat just one kernel at a time, move it around in your mouth, and get the full taste out of it, then take another single kernel. Stay with this one kernel at a time, savoring until the bag is half gone. Then throw the rest away. If you feel guilty about throwing away half of the popcorn, remember the simple motto that "it is better for it to go to waste than to go to your waist."

You will find that it took you longer to eat the half bag on day three than the whole bag on day one—probably twice as long—and you will find that you enjoyed it twice as much, and that you feel better about having eaten it, and that you just feel better. (Perhaps twice as good?)

It is important to recognize that a lot of American culture works against the quality-over-quantity, smaller-is-better mentality. Fast-food chains encourage us to "supersize" everything, and people walk (or waddle) out of gas stations carrying sixty-four-ounce jugs of soda. It's a little better in Europe, where you might go to a British tea party and savor a tiny crumpet or stir afternoon tea with a miniature spoon before sipping it from a dainty cup. Or you might go to France and get a petite, six-ounce soda can out of a vending machine.

The interesting thing is that smaller bites generate bigger flavor because there's room in your mouth to move the morsel around and to taste it with more parts of your tongue. It just feels better—not unlike a large spacious room with minimal fine furniture that seems more pleasant and tranquil than a cramped room stuffed with mediocre furnishings and knickknacks.

Along with eating less, you will eat more slowly and better. You will begin to eat less like an animal and more like an artist.

Along with eating less, you will eat more slowly and better. You will begin to eat less like an animal and more like an artist.

There is a "second taste," a second wave of flavor that comes if we take smaller bites and chew and savor them a little longer. Almost as when a cow chews its cud, the well-masticated morsels yield a smooth, blended aftertaste from each bite just before we send it off toward the appreciative stomach.

One aspect of this more artistic eating is the ability to focus on one bite of one food at a time rather than mixing things into a large artless mass in the mouth. Having a small amount in the mouth just works better, like a small load in a clothes washer; there's more space to tumble and taste the food.

WHO IS WINNING: YOU OR YOUR APPETITE?

It is so interesting to sit in a restaurant or an airport or a fast-food place and watch people eat. I always watch to see who is winning—the person or the appetite. Usually the appetite is winning.

When the appetite is winning, people eat quickly. Their fork is loading up the next bite the second they get the previous bite in their mouth. Their eyes are darting around from plate to fork and over to the bread and then to their drink, like they are protecting their food as they gulp and guzzle it down.

Even in very nice restaurants, you see a lot of appetites winning. The bites are big and too rapid in their succession. It's a subconscious thing; the person may be carrying on a conversation and using good table manners, but if you look closely, the appetite is winning.

It's so refreshing when you see someone who is winning over the appetite, who is bridling, who is reining in the horse and thus enjoying it more. I like to watch

> I like to watch someone taking his or her time, smelling and savoring the food, arranging a small bite on the fork then setting the fork down between bites and chewing slowly. These people have a much calmer demeanor.

someone taking his or her time, smelling and savoring the food, arranging a small bite on the fork then setting the fork down between bites and chewing slowly. These people have a much calmer demeanor. There is a look of control and peace and awareness of what is around them as well as what is on their plate, and these people never seem to be seriously overweight.

We need to learn to ask ourselves as we are eating, "Who is the master here, and who is the servant? Who is winning: me or my appetite?"

The cool thing is that you don't need a fancy restaurant and fine china and silver in order to eat in a refined (and diet-conscious) way. It's all in the head. Example: someone sitting on a New York park bench in the sun on an unseasonably warm winter day, head back, taking in the rays, and eating, very slowly and thoughtfully, a sauerkraut hot dog on a Kaiser roll; he is the master, his appetite the servant.

How about the phrase "healthy appetite"? Perhaps we need to redefine what that means. Sometimes we picture it as a really hungry person wolfing down his food. Actually, that is an unhealthy appetite—an appetite that is winning and that is doing damage to the body.

A better definition of a healthy appetite is a controlled appetite, a bridled appetite that goes only as fast and only as far as the rider wants it to go and that enjoys every step or every bite. That kind of appetite is truly healthy, both physically and spiritually, and will serve us well for both the short term and the long.

Watch people eat and see what you think. And then watch yourself eat. Make it a beautiful thing. Over time, it will make you a beautiful thing, too.

Practice the art of eating half as much twice as slowly. As you do, you will begin to notice a higher level of awareness, of enjoyment, and of discernment about what you eat. However, it will still be hard and will still require discipline. I have some additional tips that can help, and one of the best and the simplest of them will be the subject of the next chapter.

CHAPTER 4

MAKE WATER YOUR ALLY

One of the simplest ways to eat less food is to make less room for it by filling your stomach up with the beautiful, clearing, cleansing, lubricating, hydrating, zero-calorie substance we call water.

Doctors and nutritionists have been telling us for decades that most of us need to drink more water—six to ten good-size glasses of it every day. Not liquids—water. It's hard to drink that much unless we're sipping away pretty steadily.

One thing that can help you halve your quantity intake is the habit of always drinking a big, clear glass of water before you eat anything. Drinking a full glass before each meal results in two good, simple results:

1. More water.
2. Less food.

One thing that can help you halve your quantity intake is the habit of always drinking a big, clear glass of water before you eat anything.

Both are accomplished by the simple resolution that becomes a habit: "Before I eat anything—meals *or* snacks—I will drink a full glass of water." Filling your stomach part of the way up with water is the simplest conceivable way to make less room in there for food. And staying fully hydrated (something very few of us do consistently) makes you feel better in all sorts of ways.

If you want to experiment a little and focus on how good water feels to your body, wait until a moment when you are quite thirsty (after exercise, perhaps, or first thing in the morning, or maybe when you get up in the night) and then drink a couple of glasses of cold water. Then lie down, relax, close your eyes, and feel the hydration flowing through your body. If you concentrate, you'll feel the water radiating out toward your extremities, refreshing, regenerating, replenishing, and renewing every cell.

What a deal! It keeps you from eating more, and it helps your body digest what you do eat better, use the food's nutrients more efficiently, and get them distributed more effectively out to your cells.

More water really is the perfect complement to less food all day long. Get a good water bottle that you like the look and feel of and carry it around with you. Have it with you in the car, set it on your desk, keep it near when you're watching TV or reading at home. Clean and fill it often. Let sipping become a habit.

It's the easiest thing in the world to monitor yourself to make sure that you are always fully hydrated. You'll be going to the bathroom more often, and your urine will be nice and clear. If you're not going several times a day and if your urine is yellow, you're not drinking enough.

If you are having a hard time remembering to drink water, try getting a jump on it by drinking two or three full glasses first thing in the morning as you get up and brush your teeth or do your hair or take your meds. Many report that filling up with water first thing gets them feeling hydrated and ready to go for the day.

Wow! Talk about a simple key to the eat-half diet! Just drink more. It also helps your blood pressure *and* (this is the amazing thing) it somehow makes you feel more relaxed, more calm, and even more optimistic.

The best things in life are free, and one of the very best free things is water!

FIGHT THE IMPULSE

One other thing water can do for you is combat "impulse eating." Retailers thrive on impulse purchasing: shoppers who can't resist bargain-price items carefully placed where the eye glances and the hand can reach. Most of us eat like impulse purchasers shop. When we walk past food or notice food lying somewhere on the counter or in the drawer or on the shelf, we grab it and slap it into our mouths. Just a little, of course, but it adds up. Some call it "grazing" because it's a lot like what horses do: just nibbling all the time. There's food all around us in our homes, so it can be a bite here and a bite there, not even counting the full-fledged snacks. We eat what's in front of us or around us for the same reason George Leigh Mallory said he climbed Everest: "Because it's there."[3]

The problem with impulse purchasing or impulse eating is that it lets your appetite win—just in little pieces, but those small bites combine and multiply, and appetite wins while you lose (and *gain*). This has always been a tactic or a strategy in war and in selling and in sports: chipping away . . . a yard or two at a time . . . a foot in the door . . . slipping in under the radar. Little bites or nibbles can be so tiny that they don't seem to matter. But that is the subtle, seductive strategy of appetite: it claims victory over us one little innocent bite at a time.

> The problem with impulse purchasing or impulse eating is that it lets your appetite win—just in little pieces, but those small bites combine and multiply, and appetite wins while you lose (and *gain*).

One way to bridle that appetite, to get rid of the grazing habit, is to sip water instead. Keep a water bottle close and replace the grazing habit with the sipping habit. Fill up on the water that helps you instead of the food that hurts you.

It's helpful to think of your appetite as a horse. It wants to graze all the time. It is in the habit of putting its head down and nibbling. But you are the rider! You have the reins! You can pull that horse's head up every time he tries for a bite, and pretty soon, you can break his grazing habit. Let him drink from the stream, but do not let him eat from the field.

The only way to beat the grazing habit is to decide in advance to put nothing but water into your mouth between the meals and the one or two snacks you've chosen. Rein your appetite into complete submission on this. Show it who's boss. And let water be your ally!

CHAPTER 5

FIVE PER FORTNIGHT (FINDING THE EXERCISE YOU LOVE)

Putting less (and better) food into your body, and more water, is going to make your body work better. But you've still got to make your body work!

Should it be a chore, a task, a constant struggle to force this work to happen—to force your body to exercise? Does it have to be something you hate doing but keep motivating yourself to do anyway for your own good, like taking cod liver oil?

Exercising, like eating, should be one of the natural and simple and pure joys of life. It should feel good while you're doing it as well as when you're through, and it should be a way of rewarding yourself, not a way of punishing yourself.

> Exercising, like eating, should be one of the natural and simple and pure joys of life. It should feel good while you're doing it as well as when you're through.

The key is to find your form of exercise, to find the exercise you love, the one that makes your body smile while it's sweating out that pore-cleaning water and pumping those endorphins around through your expanded lungs and your healthier cardiovascular system.

For me, it's tennis. It used to be jogging, but now it's tennis: singles, without breaks between games, so that it's aerobic. For my spouse, it's the bike: the road bike if the weather is good, the stationery one at home if it's not. For my daughter, it's running; for my son, it's basketball. For my friend, it's the aerobic yoga class at the gym that has a good nursery for her two preschoolers. For another friend, it's the StairMaster while he reads the morning paper every day. For yet another friend, it's early-morning lap swimming.

THE GOOD ADDICTION

For each of these people, and for myself, our chosen form of exercise has become a *good addiction*. You can (and should) get totally hooked on the habit of exercise. I can't *not* play tennis. If I go for more than two or three days without a good match, I feel logy and heavy . . . and I also feel stressed and nervous. If I'm traveling and staying somewhere without a court or an opponent, I have to run or bike or go to a gym (though I don't like it nearly as much) in order to satisfy my endorphin need.

I'm always looking forward to my next match and usually reflecting back happily on the last one (though not so much if I lost). When I tore a knee ligament a few years ago and couldn't play (or run), I nearly went nuts until I found a trainer who convinced me that the injury was actually an opportunity to work on my upper body strength, which would make me a stronger and better player when my knee healed.

What I'm saying here is simply that you've got to find a physical passion of some kind—a form of exercise that you love. You don't need to instantly love it. It can take a little time to get into something, to get good enough at it that it's enjoyable, and to get hooked on the way it makes you feel. If you don't know what your physical passion might be, start trying things until you find one.

The point is that we all need an "output" to go with our improved "input." Disciplining ourselves with regard to our input into our bodies—less and better food and more water—has to be accompanied by the passion and rigor of the output of our exercise. One side is working on the quality and quantity of the calories we put in, and the other side is developing the most enjoyable and beneficial way of burning and sweating them out!

Earlier generations didn't have to think or strategize nearly as much about the input or the output. Their hard physical work was the output, and it was usually so strenuous that it burned up all the input, no matter what it was. But in our age of technology and desk or keyboard jobs, we clearly need a well-thought-out and carefully implemented strategy for both input and output. The point is that it can be an enjoyable strategy!

> One side is working on the quality and quantity of the calories we put in, and the other side is developing the most enjoyable and beneficial way of burning and sweating them out!

Depending on the type of exercise you choose, you may be able to do it almost every day, or it may be something you're only able to do two or three times a week (which is about the minimum frequency that will do much good).

Actually, the minimum ought to be five per fortnight. I like the British term "fortnight"—two weeks—because it gives more flexibility. Maybe you only get to your chosen exercise twice one week, so you crank it up to at least three the next week to meet the minimum of five per fortnight.

The trouble is, of course, that it is probably not possible to play tennis, or swim, or bike, or do whatever your chosen recreation is every day. And our bodies do need at least a twenty-minute taste of aerobic exercise every day in order to feel tuned and trimmed.

So expand your positive physical addiction by walking or jogging or going on a treadmill or elliptical or stationary bike every day that you don't do your "sport." Find a formula that works for you—read or watch the news while you ride a stationary bike, take the dog to walk or jog with you, put a treadmill in front of the TV and never watch without running. Spend the time and the thought it takes to figure out your own daily discipline and fortnightly five, and once you have them, never let them go!

Find it! Do it! Love it! Lose it!

CHAPTER 6

FASTING AND "SLOWING"

For centuries, for millennia, forever, fasting has been associated with mental and spiritual clarity and with a cleansing and purging of the physical body. It can also help with the development of discipline that will make the Half Diet really work.

As hard as it is to divide the food on your plate and eat only half of it, it is even harder (twice as hard?) to eat none of it at all. Periodic fasting recalibrates your appetite, your sense of self-control, and even the size of your stomach.

In order to formulate my specific fasting challenge, let me define the terms and the timetable. For our purposes here, let's define fasting as going completely without food or drink (except water) for twenty-four hours—essentially missing two meals and going from dinner on one day to dinner on the next day without eating anything in between.

Fasting once a month for twenty-four hours is a fairly widespread practice. Mormons call the first Sunday of the month "Fast Sunday," and similar patterns are found in other religions around the world. Hindus, for example, often fast with each new moon.

Here are ten (mostly beneficial) results of a once-a-month fast:

1. It clears out and rests your whole physical system.

2. It focuses your mind. You will think with new clarity about many things.

3. It enhances your "gratitude attitude," or your ability to feel and express thanks or appreciation (not just for food but for life at large).

4. It makes you humbler and more aware of your dependence on nature, on the earth, on God.

5. It fine-tunes your priorities and makes you more capable of separating the things that really matter from the things that really don't.

6. (Being candid) It can make you feel nasty and short tempered.

7. (Being candid again) It can make you feel too weak to do anything.

8. It calms your mind and slows you down.

9. It gives you perspective as you think about and plan the month ahead.

10. It makes the Half Diet seem easier. (After fasting, eating half seems like a lovely luxury rather than a disciplined deprivation.)

Two negatives out of ten isn't bad, and numbers 6 and 7 tend to fade as you get more used to fasting.

SLOWING TIME DOWN

Let's focus on number 8 for a minute, partly because I like the play on words in "fasting causes slowing." Think of some phrases we hear often these days (maybe that we say often): "If I could just slow time down a little," "There are not enough hours in the day," "So many tasks, so little time," or "If I could clone myself, maybe I could get everything done." Of these frequently heard sentiments, one of them may actually be feasible—the first one. We will never have more hours, more time, or a second self, but it actually is possible to slow time down a little.

When we get stressed and frantic and run around madly, trying to get everything done, time seems to speed up just to frustrate us more. But sometimes, when we are calm and introspective, time seems to slow a bit and become more peaceful in its passing. One of the best ways I know to obtain a peaceful mind is to fast. During a fast, you feel less nervous energy, less tendency to rush or to worry about details. Fasting makes it easier to have perspective, to see the big picture, to focus in on what really matters. As this happens, time seems to slow down. Even a slightly clearer mind and slightly slower time are well worth the little bit of hunger you'll feel during a regular monthly fast.

As a matter of fact, the hunger itself is a good thing, too. While you are fasting, hunger confirms that you are, at that moment, the master over your appetite for food. Your appetite says eat. You say no. Hunger confirms that you have won.

Some Half Dieters have come to love the feeling that monthly fasting gives them so much that they also do a partial weekly fast, skipping breakfast every Sunday and eating nothing until a late lunch.

A little hunger, as I said, is not a bad thing. It enhances our sense of gratitude and our empathy for the third of the people on our planet who feel hunger all day and who go to bed with it every night. *And*, if

> Sometimes, when we are calm and introspective, time seems to slow a bit and become more peaceful in its passing. One of the best ways I know to obtain a peaceful mind is to fast.

> A little hunger is not a bad thing. It enhances our sense of gratitude and our empathy for the third of the people on our planet who feel hunger all day and who go to bed with it every night.

you are a person of spiritual inclination, fasting seems to be the perfect accompaniment to prayer, making spiritual contact with a higher power seem more direct and more natural.

THE ACID TEST: APPLYING THE HALF DIET TO HOLIDAY EATING

For so many people, holidays and vacations have become a time for state-of-the-art overeating. Yet, ironically, celebrations, feasts, and holidays can actually be the best times to implement this diet.

The Half Diet is really, at its core, about enjoying food more, so what better times could there be to employ it than at special, celebratory times of the year?

The real trick is to change our assumptions. The old assumption is that the more we eat, the more we enjoy, but we know that isn't really true. There is no correlation between the quantity of food we eat and the quantity of joy we feel. In fact, there is usually an inverse relationship. The more we eat, the less joy we find.

The Half Diet is not about what we shouldn't eat. It is about controlling quantity in a way that allows us to focus more on quality and on the joy of every (small) bite. It's not about what we shouldn't do but about what we should do to maximize both the joy of eating and the joy of our bodies—and, ultimately, the joy of our lives. And joy is all about quality and higher consciousness and greater awareness and perspective. It is, in other words (using the food metaphor), all about sipping and savoring.

Holidays are simply the perfect time to employ the basic Half Diet principle of eating half as much twice as slowly. Those who are into the diet and have begun to reap its rewards will see the wonderful and plentiful food of vacations and celebrations through a different lens: the healthy things will look good to you, and the unhealthy ones will look bad.

Remember that one of the key underlying principles of the diet is that when you cut your quantity to half and hold it at half for many consecutive days, your body, failing to get the greater quantity, will start asking you for greater quality. The main job of your appetite is to get the nutrients into your body that it requires to function, and if your appetite can get you to eat enough junk to get the necessary nutrients, it will do so. But if you enforce the eat-half discipline for long enough, your appetite will realize that the only way to get its nutrients from half the quantity is to demand more quality. You will start craving fruit and vegetables and other wholesome and healthy foods and will *gradually* start loathing the greasy, heavy, or refined junk foods. You want this to begin happening before big holidays, especially Thanksgiving and Christmas, so start now, recommit, and have your appetites in training before the next holiday hits.

Try to visualize yourself surrounded by food at parties, at dinners, and even just walking around your festive house. Visualize yourself walking past food and not picking it up unless it is mealtime or snack time (three half meals, two half snacks, nothing else).

Visualize yourself drinking a tall glass of water before each meal or snack. Visualize yourself eating what you want at those meals and snacks, but only half of it. Visualize yourself eating very slowly, with small bites, smelling and savoring the food, and sipping whatever you drink. Visualize yourself eating the quality food that lends itself to small bites and savoring. Visualize yourself finding time to slip away for a walk or a jog or whatever your chosen form of exercise is. Visualize a lovely celebration and family time full of flavor, of awareness, of perspective, and of the kind of bridling that fills you with love!

THE RESET OR REBOOT OF A NAP

Another way to reset your psyche is to take a brief power nap. Yes, yes, diet books are supposed to be about eating and not about sleeping. But as you are finding out, this diet is about much more than

Did you know that people who take a semiregular brief nap in the afternoon or early evening have a 37 percent lower incidence of heart attacks?

food. It is about maximizing our time here on earth—physically, mentally, and spiritually. And guess what? Sleeping is a big part of our time here on earth and deserves some mention.

Did you know that people who take a semiregular brief nap in the afternoon or early evening have a 37 percent lower incidence of heart attacks? Here are some excerpts (with my commentary) from a *Newsweek* article.[5]

> Researchers at the Harvard School of Public Health and the University of Athens Medical School have just released findings from a large study that shows how mid-day napping reduces one's chance of coronary mortality by more than a third. So go ahead and nap—a short daily snooze might ward off a heart attack later in life.

The study looked at 23,681 individuals living in Greece who had no personal history of coronary heart disease, stroke, or cancer when they first volunteered. What they found was pretty amazing.

> More than six years later, the exemplary nappers, men and women who napped at least three times per week for an average of at least 30 minutes, had a 37 percent lower coronary mortality risk than those who took no siestas. The so-so nappers, who only snoozed occasionally, showed a reduction in mortality of about 12 percent. That sounds good, but it's not statistically significant, say researchers. The lesson: if you're going to nap, be ambitious and do it several times a week.

The fact is that the culture of some parts of the world, including the tradition of taking naps, is just plain healthy!

> Siestas are common in Mediterranean regions like southern Italy and southern Greece, as well as several Latin American countries, all of which happen to have low mortality rates from coronary disease. Several of those areas are famed for a Mediterranean diet that makes heavy use of heart-friendly foods like olive oil. "But people are careless there," says Dimitrios Trichopoulos, a pro-

fessor of epidemiology at the Harvard School of Public Health and one of the napping study's authors. "They don't exercise and health care is mediocre. Yet they have lower coronary mortality rates. It couldn't just be the olive oil. That's why we started exploring the effects of the siesta."

And it's not just the Harvard and University of Athens studies that show the benefits of napping:

NASA sleep researchers have found that a nap of 26 minutes can boost performance by as much as 34 percent. A 2006 study from the Stanford University School of Medicine found that napping resulted in improved mood, increased alertness, and reduced lapses in performance among doctors and nurses.

How about that?

Studies indicate that twenty minutes of sleep in the afternoon provide more rest than twenty minutes more sleep in the morning (though the last two hours of morning sleep have special benefits of their own). The body seems to be designed for this, as most people's bodies naturally become more tired in the afternoon, about eight hours after we wake up.

Lots people feel a midafternoon slump in mood and alertness, especially after a poor night of sleep. Many believe this slump is caused by eating a heavy lunch. However, in reality, this occurs because we were meant to have a midafternoon nap.

Many experts advise people keep the nap between fifteen and thirty minutes, as sleeping longer gets you into deeper stages of sleep, from which it's more difficult to awaken.

EVIDENCE

Several lines of evidence, including the universal tendency of toddlers and the elderly to nap in the afternoon and the afternoon nap of siesta cultures, have led sleep researchers to the same conclusion: nature intended that we take a nap in the middle of the day. This biological readiness to fall asleep midafternoon coincides with a slight drop in body temperature and occurs regardless of whether we eat lunch at all. It is present even in good sleepers who are well rested.

So there is lots of well-documented evidence of the benefits of a little nap in the afternoon, but it is disregarded by most of us because of two rather overpowering feelings:

1. I am too busy or too occupied (by work or by kids) to nap.

2. I can't just lie down and go to sleep. My body doesn't work that way.

And although John F. Kennedy, Winston Churchill, Albert Einstein, Thomas Edison, Johannes Brahms, Napoleon Bonaparte, Leonardo da Vinci, and a long list of other historical figures reportedly loved to catnap, many Americans still associate napping with people who are lazy, stupid, or don't have the right stuff.

Eating and sleeping (and how we do both of them) are two of the four most important things we do for our bodies. (The other two are exercising and breathing.)

And besides, you may be saying, "Wait a minute. I would love to take a nap every day, but who are these people? Don't they have kids? Don't they have jobs? How do you just take a nap in the afternoon?" Napping at work is not the norm. A stigma is attached to it. It's okay for people to go out to exercise at noontime, but not to nap.

Others will say, "Yes, yes, I understand that naps are good, but I just can't lie down and fall asleep. My mind won't turn off that easily. I would just be lying there and thinking about the things I should be doing, and the whole thing would be frustrating. I would feel like I was wasting time."

So there are lots of excuses and reasons why naps won't work, but remember that eating and sleeping (and how we do both of them) are two of the four most important things we do for our bodies. (The other two are exercising and breathing, which we talk about in other chapters.) So don't dismiss the nap habit before you have thought about it and tried it.

Lots of moms find, busy and overwhelmed though they are, some opportunities for a little nap. Moms with young children may find a few minutes while their kids are napping. Moms with school-age kids may find a brief opportunity before the kids come home. People at work may find a place where they can lie down for a few moments or even rest their head on the desk like we used to do in the school library.

A KEY AND A SKILL

Here is the key: napping, like eating slowly and eating half, is a skill you can learn and a taste you can acquire! The first few times you try it, you may not get to sleep or if you do, you may wake up groggy, or disoriented, or wake up too late or so tired you wish you hadn't tried it. But you can learn how to nap in a way that is beneficial.

You can actually program your mind to wake you up in ten minutes, or twenty, or whatever you have. You can look at the dial of your watch and say, "The minute hand is on the three right now, and I will wake up when it is on the six." It may not work the first time, but it will soon. You can learn to turn off your mind and go mentally blank and drift quickly into sleep. You can think of a little nap as the reset button that resyncs your brain and your energy. You can do all this with a little practice.

Don't make napping a chore, and don't feel like you have to schedule it every day. Try to find the right moment two or three times a week and let it grow on you. If you don't get to sleep in your designated little time, don't worry. Rest is almost as good, and maybe you will drift off next time. Just get as comfortable as you can and try to completely relax.

Some find that they have to relax their body one part at a time, first concentrating on relaxing their neck muscles, then their hands and feet, then their legs and arms, etc. Try different things. Find your own way to turn off your body and your mind for a few minutes, and let the sleep come or not come.

Many people, particularly those in creative fields, find that they do their best work early in the morning and late at night. They are the quietest times, the most beautiful. Often we want to be both a "lark" and an "owl" so we can take advantage of both of these productive periods.

But people usually consider them to be mutually exclusive and assume that they can't have them both.

However, with the addition of an afternoon nap, you can! Some find that if they can take a little nap in the late afternoon, just when they are running down and getting drowsy because they got up early, they get recharged and feel great for the evening, even the late evening.

> As you get a little better at the art of napping, clearer thoughts and better ideas will start to come to you, often right after a little nap.

Different people have different needs, different lifestyles, different ways of living each day. But most people can benefit from learning to take a nap a few afternoons a week.

It's worth fooling around with. It's worth a little experimentation. It's worth the ten or twenty minutes you find to try it. There is no downside and lots of upsides to trying. And it fits extremely well with the Half Diet. It is way of training your body and your mind to serve your will.

As you get a little better at the art of napping, clearer thoughts and better ideas will start to come to you, often right after a little nap. Your head will be clearer, and the Spirit will speak to you a bit easier. A nap will give you that little recharge you need to relish rather than resist the rest of the day.

CHAPTER 7

REPAIRING THE BREACH (GIVING AWAY THE HALF YOU DON'T EAT)

You may think your desire to lose weight is the only justification you need to live by the Half Diet. But if you want it, there is a deeper and higher level of motivation that may also help.

Four thousand years ago, the prophet Isaiah foresaw our day. He predicted and warned about many things, none more graphic and haunting than his 58th chapter, in which he speaks of the growing gap or "breach" between the rich and the poor.

Today, we live in this prophecy. Each year, the richest in our world get richer and the poor get poorer. The richest 5 percent of the planet's population control and possess more than half of the world's resources, while the poorest 33 percent have only 1 percent of the world's wealth. This third of the world goes to bed hungry each night and sleeps on dirt floors.

As the breach gets wider, it destroys the happiness of both extremes. The poorest of the poor face insurmountable problems of hunger, thirst, disease, and lack of education. The richest of the rich (which, on a relative global scale, certainly includes most Americans) face the opposite, but potentially equally devastating (especially to kids), problems of boredom, indifference, instant gratification, attitudes of entitlement, and lack of appreciation.

The gap or the breach is the enemy that undermines both sides. No wonder Isaiah challenged us to be, each in our own way, "repairers of the breach."

HOW IS THE BREACH CONNECTED TO THE DIET?

So what has any of this to do with the Half Diet? Well, let's go back again to the "kids are starving in Africa" cliché so many of our mothers used to get us to clean our plates. While the cause and effect may not be quite as direct as Mom implied, children in Ethiopia and Haiti *are* starving, and it is not completely beyond our capacity to help. Remember that no matter how wide the breach is, you become one of its repairers if you close the gap even one microsliver by feeding one poor child.

In addition, making a small effort in that direction can have a positive psychological effect on our ability to observe and follow the physical Diet. It completes the circle, in a way. As we eat half, we give the other half to someone who benefits as much from having it as we benefit from giving it up.

It completes the circle, in a way. As we eat half, we give the other half to someone who benefits as much from having it as we benefit from giving it up.

Relatively easy ways to accomplish this include sponsoring a third-world child for about thirty dollars a month or making small, regular donations to a local soup kitchen or shelter. Doing something like this will complete the loop and add a very interesting and beneficial form of motivation to your effort to consistently eat half.

Make your eat-less-and-give-more formula as mathematically accurate as you can. You won't spend half as much money on the food you eat with the diet, because as the quality of your food goes up, some of it will cost more. But make up a food budget for a week or a month while you are eating half. Then compare it with an estimate of what you spent before and find a way to give roughly the difference to those who are hungry.

Don't fall victim to the old "realistic" excuse about the problem being so big and global that you are obviously incapable of making a dent in it. Environmentalists don't recycle because they think they can rid the whole world of pollution; neither do they avoid aerosol cans because they think they can single-handedly fix the ozone hole. Instead, each one does what he does because it is his tiny part and because it is the right thing to do and because it makes him a stronger, better person.

We can be like that—like the beach walker who came upon a vast mass of beached starfish and started throwing them back one at a time. An amused critic passed by and said, "There are too many. You'll never make a difference." The man threw another one out into deep water and said, "I made a difference to that one."[4] He also made a difference to himself, to his character, and to his motivation—the same kind of difference you will make as you eat half and give half away.

Giving half and repairing the breach can give us empathy and help us see things as others see them. As we adopt some of the appreciation and the awareness of those we help, our own lives become richer and our motivation for the Half Diet grows stronger.

CHAPTER 8

POETRY
(LIVING IN AND
SEEING THE MOMENT)

Where are we going with this one—poetry as part of a diet? Yes! And it's not as weird as you think. Here's the concept: This diet is all about awareness and sensitivity: being aware of the quality and amount of what you eat—appreciating it, tasting it, sipping and savoring it. To improve and perfect our ability to do this, we have to work on improving and perfecting our ability to be aware and sensitive in a broader and more general sense. Awareness and sensitivity are qualities that can be developed, skills that can be learned and practiced.

There is no better way to do that than to attempt some poetry! Have no fear; this is private poetry that no one will critique or judge. In fact, no one will even see it unless you happen to write one you think is so good that you just have to show it to somebody.

Think about the process of writing a poem; if you've never tried it, imagine what you think that process might be. First, you have to really notice something—become acutely aware of how it looks or sounds or feels or smells or tastes and how it makes you feel. Second, you have to hold that image in your mind, to visualize it. Third, you have to discipline yourself to actually sit down and try to describe it, to write about it.

> The skills and perspectives you develop by trying to write poetry will help you become better at the diet.

The awareness and visualization and discipline of the Half Diet are so similar to this practice. And the skills and perspectives you develop by trying to write poetry will help you become better at the diet.

Poetry can be about anything you notice and appreciate. Try to write some poems about your own body, about your appreciation for some of its particular functions or form, about your visualization of how you want it to become, about the miraculous nature of its ability to assimilate high-quality foods and turn them into energy and muscle.

Use visualization to heal and improve your body. Write poems about health and vigor. "See" yourself the way you want to be. Imagine, in vivid detail, your arteries carrying blood or your lungs assimilating oxygen or your antibodies warding off infection. Use poetry as a way of capturing these positive images.

The type of thinking required to support and enhance the Half Diet is both analytic and artistic, part science and part creativity. Writing poetry (even bad attempts at poetry) provides the best way to mentally summon this combination!

THE CHALLENGE IS TO TRY IT

Here's the challenge: get a notebook or diary or some kind of little blank book that you can keep track of and write something in it every day. It might just be one line of a poem, or a description of something you noticed that you can incorporate into a poem later. Some days, you will be inspired and write a complete poem, but the commitment to write something every day will cause you to be aware and to be looking and noticing more than usual.

Try thinking about where you are, what you can see or hear, what you are feeling, what your body is doing while you are eating. While you are sipping, savoring, and smelling your half portion of food, use the slowness of those moments to reflect a little, to let thoughts come into your mind, to try to be in the moment as you taste and appreciate your food. Open your book and write what you feel. If a day slips by and you have not written a line, try naming the day. Think back to something you noticed or enjoyed, something you felt, and come up with a poetic name for that moment.

Poetry doesn't have to rhyme or follow some particular meter or structure. Just use the most descriptive and clear words you can think of to describe what you are seeing or feeling. Use as few words as you can. Choose the words in the same way you are learning to choose your food, with quality being more important than quantity.

Here, as examples, are four poems written by implementers of the Half Diet. None of them will win a prize, but writing them was helpful in noticing, helpful in slowing down, helpful in being in the present, and thus helpful in dieting. You can do just as well!

Liquid Light

The clear glass fills with clear water,
Bubbling up, cold from tap to rim, catching light.
Then to my lips, a sip, a swallow,
Then a pulsing river flowing down,
Cooling and cleansing, pooling in the center of me,
Then trickling out through my tributaries to legs and arms
Some percolates back up, through another part of my neck
To cool and clear my brain.

Aerobics, First Day

A strange mood prompts me to see
if I can survive an hour.
By happenstance I get in an advanced class.
The instructor is a girl shaped like a
Silver stovepipe,
Insufficient flesh to have curves
And wearing shiny grey tights.
Even her hoarse voice is metallic,
Is she bionic?
Because she never stops,
Never tires or frowns or moans,
Never even sweats.
I do all of those things.
Each provides a modicum of relief.
The music pulses loud against
The glitter and glass.
It's a disco really; strobe lights
Would look right in place,
Glistening bodies and leg warmers.
A new phenomenon combining
Narcissism and vanity
But a more obtainable pride
Than most
And not all bad.
(But don't ask my body!)

A Sky Like That

Leaving the office one routine day
glanced up
and beheld
the glory bursts of heaven's sun

behind the gray, receding storm clouds.

Late March after a day-long snow

now, air winter crisp,

clarion clear.

Sky's pure, pale, delicate blue

(since it's so new) and the still-gray retreating clouds

with edges dazzling white,

giving away the presence of the sun.

They still try to hide—

Had I been all day in a great museum

Unseen—studying works of masters

my reaction would have been the same

walking out . . .

"This is beauty"

and all works of man

fail to compare.

Early Light

Looked out this morning early

light

long before usual

white round snow, white round moon, blue sky, gold only

along east rim

even light,

with no dominating source

part moon, part dawn, part snow-earth reflection

stereophonic light

comes from everywhere

bathes all the air with just enough illumination

to see

and be

moved

by its beauty.

So just do it—try your hand at a poem or two. It is part of the Half Diet, and you can do it!

The perspective that you gain by attempting a poem is often a lot like hitting the reset button, and life looks a little fresher, a little clearer.

CHAPTER 9

THE HORSE AND THE BRIDLE

Horse riders and horse lovers know how strong those magnificent animals are. They outweigh us by a factor of five or six to one, but that's just the beginning. Their tendon and muscle connections give them a leverage that probably doubles their weight advantage. You may already know that if you have been literally thrown across the barn by a horse that was startled and lifted its head.

Because of their strength and their beauty, horses have been used by man for countless things ranging from toil to pleasure. They have also been used since antiquity for one of the most apt metaphors in history.

"We put bits in the horses' mouths," said James, an apostle of the New Testament, "that they may obey us; and we turn about their whole body."[6] To become "perfect men," he said, we must be "able also to bridle" our bodies,[7] our expressions, our appetites. Other ancient scripture warns (and promises), "See that ye bridle all your passions, that ye may be filled with love."[8]

One reason the horse is such a perfect metaphor is that horses are extraordinary, remarkable, and beautiful creatures than can serve us in ways that are exciting and thrilling as well as useful. There is nothing quite like a horse at full gallop, especially if you are on its back, moving with it and feeling its grace and power.

If you focus only on the danger that a horse potentially poses—thinking only about its strength and potential to hurt you—the horse could begin to seem like an enemy, something you need to fight and subdue. One way to be sure that a horse does not hurt you would be to tranquilize it or drug it to neutralize its strength. And the way to absolutely guarantee that a horse will not hurt you would be to kill it. But what a foolish and cowardly approach that would be; it would deny the beauty and the usefulness of the horse.

> Until we put the bit of our own control between the teeth of our urges and instincts, these appetites can injure us, wound our destiny, and throw us off the path of our dreams and our goals.

So it is with our passions and our appetites. These are not things we should want to kill or to medicate out of our lives. They are not our enemies but our energies. They can be our motivators rather than our masters and a thrill to ride rather than a threat to ruin.

But only with the bridle! Until we put the bit of our own control between the teeth of our urges and instincts, these appetites can injure us, wound our destiny, and throw us off the path of our dreams and our goals.

The last thing we should want to do with our appetites—for food, or for sex, or for any of life's gifts—is dull them, subdue them, tie them up, or hobble them so they lose their beauty and strength and passion. We do not want to kill these things, because they are not our enemies. Rather, we should bridle our appetite, harness it, and control it to work with us and for us instead of on us and against us.

Your brain is the bridle, and your mental commitment to eat half as much twice as slowly is the bit that can gradually come to feel natural and accepted in the mouth!

As you eat half, twice as slowly and with twice the appreciation and en-joyment, keep the horse in mind: think of your soul as the rider and your will as the bridle. If it helps, try to visualize me handing you the bridle, helping you slip it over the horse's head, helping you get the bit between its teeth, putting the reins in your hand, telling you to show the horse who is boss, helping you stay in control, and showing you how to enjoy the ride.

CHAPTER 10

REVIEW OF THE PRINCIPLES AND PRACTICES OF THE PHYSICAL DIET

I n this chapter, let's take a look back and review what we have covered so far in the physical part of the Half Diet. It is important to have the principles and practices well in your mind both to implement the body-diet and to help comprehend the mind-diet and spirit-diet that are still to come.

Sixteen simple principles of the physical diet:

1. Natural foods, in all their variety, are good for the body.

2. Appetite, while it can direct us to the food our body needs, doesn't know when to quit.

3. We normally eat about twice as much as we need.

4. By eating half of that—half as much as usual (and holding the line and doing it consistently)—we will gradually gravitate toward food

that is twice as good (because our bodies, denied quantity, will demand quality).

5. By eating half as quickly, we can enjoy food twice as much.

6. The more sensual attention we pay to eating, the more pleasurable it becomes.

7. Disciplining both the amount we eat and the pace at which we eat further enhances the pleasure.

8. Our bodies need more water as much as they need less food. A stomach that is full of water will ask for and be satisfied with less food.

9. Allowing the whole digestive system to shut down and rest periodically (through fasting) can cleanse, rejuvenate, and recalibrate capacity.

10. Mental and spiritual awareness are heightened and sharpened by fasting.

11. Disciplining the "output" of exercise is as important as regulating the "input" of eating.

12. With some effort and attention, everyone can find a form of physical exercise he or she loves. Exercise, because of the endorphins it produces, can become a positive physical addiction.

13. Giving away the half we do not eat increases our motivation even as it feeds our brothers and pleases our divine Father.

14. Poetry or other artistic outlets enhance awareness, slow us down, orient us to quality, and increase our discipline.

15. Slowing down for proper rest, including regular, short naps, can improve overall wellness and productivity.

16. The horse-and-bridle metaphor can help us understand, visualize, and implement the diet.

Seven simple practices of the physical diet:

1. Eat half of each of your normal three meals a day and one or two half snacks. Nothing else.

2. Eat slowly. Sip, savor, and smell, so the half takes as long as the whole used to.

3. Drink a tall glass of water before each half meal or half snack.

4. Fast for twenty-four hours once a month.

5. Exercise aerobically (find a form you love) for at least twenty minutes every day, and participate in an actual sport at least five times each fortnight.

6. Give the equivalent of the half you don't eat to those in need.

7. Write one or more poems per week. (Write something in your awareness every day.)

Do you believe these sixteen principles? Can you implement these seven practices? Let your belief in the principles grow your motivation to implement the practices. Work at it! Don't give up! The results will be there, if they are not already. And the results you see on your scale will be just the beginning.

REDUCING IT ALL DOWN TO FIVE BAD HABITS AND FIVE GOOD HABITS

As a final simplification of the physical Half Diet (and, let's face it, we all need simplification), let's think of the whole thing as a matter of habits.

Human bodies are amazingly resilient and will withstand a lot of abuse, but some of our bad habits are wearing our bodies down and undermining our health in ways that we don't notice or recognize as clearly as we should.

And the further it goes, the harder it is to reverse.

We are not talking about alcohol or substance abuse, or about being a total couch potato, or about a diet composed entirely of junk food. People who are doing extreme, dramatic, or obvious things to destroy their bodies already know about it and don't need books like this one to point it out to them.

We are talking about less obvious things—habits we get into that gradually drag us down and wear us out and hurt our ability to feel our best and be at our best for our families. There are five of them:

1. *Chronic dehydration.* We don't drink enough. Or we drink the wrong things. Sodas and diet drinks don't rehydrate us. Most of us drink less than half of the eight glasses of water necessary to keep us hydrated. Doctors tell us that most Americans are in some stage of chronic dehydration, which undermines the health of our organs, from our skin to our digestive tract.

2. *Fast eating.* It's not just fast food that gets us; it's fast eating. The faster we shovel food in, the less well we digest it and the more we eat. Our bites are too big and too rapid. We tend to guzzle, gulp, and gorge instead of smelling, sipping, and savoring our food.

3. *Huge portions.* We live in the land of supersizing. Our drinks are too big, our entrées are too big, our plates are too big, our portions are just too big.

4. *Endless snacking.* The problem is that there is always food around us. In the cupboard, on the counter, in the fridge, in the gas station convenience store, in the fast food places we pass, in vending machines. It's usually high in salt and sugar and low in nutrients. We see it, we eat it.

5. *Too much sitting.* Eighty-five percent of Americans have jobs that are accomplished while sitting, and then we sit in our car or on a train as we commute back and forth, and then we sit on the couch and watch TV, and then we sit at our computers and do social media or answer emails. Sit, sit, sit—not exactly what our bodies were designed to do or something they are improved by.

The reason we let ourselves get away with these five bad habits is that their effects on us are very gradual. We don't just wake up one morning and find ourselves fat or run-down or sick or slow. Everything comes on us gradually. What we have to understand is the definition of "chronic." Chronic situations are those that become worse over time and that pull us down and limit our potential very slowly.

But the way to change all this is not slow or gradual. The best correction is an immediate one. The best way to break a habit is to drop it.

We can literally stop doing these five things right now!

If we recognize them and understand their insidious and damaging nature, we can find the motivation to simply stop all five, to reverse them by simply drinking more, eating more slowly, avoiding or limiting or improving the quality of snacks, sharing meals or reducing portions, and exercising or moving a little more each day.

> The way to change all this is not slow or gradual. The best correction is an immediate one. The best way to break a habit is to drop it.

The best way, of course, to break any bad habit is to substitute a good habit for it, and the antithesis of these five bad habits are the five good habits that form the core of the Half Diet:

1. *The water habit.* Drink a tall glass of water immediately before each of your three daily meals. Besides hydrating you, this fills your stomach and reduces your appetite.

2. *The slow habit.* Set your fork or spoon down on the table after each bite. This slows down your eating and causes you to enjoy a meal more while actually consuming less.

3. *The half habit.* Prepare or order whatever meal you want, but eat only half of it. If you are eating out, share your meal with your spouse or friend or take half of it home. If you are eating at home, eat exactly half of your normal portions.

4. *The snack habit.* Only snack on fruit or vegetables. Except for your three meals, do not eat anything unless it is a fruit or vegetable.

5. *The move habit.* Devote twenty minutes a day to some kind of aerobic exercise that doubles your normal heart rate. It can be something as simple as a brisk walk or time on a treadmill or a stationary bike, but do it every day.

These habits take commitment and discipline, but they can actually develop and become part of your life rather quickly! If you do something for twenty-one straight days, it becomes a habit.

Start a chart where you check off each of the five habits every day. On day one, put a "1" for each of the five that you do that day. On the second day, put a "2." If you miss a day on one of the habits, start over on your numbering for that habit. Stay with it until you get to twenty-one consecutive days on each of the five habits.

Habit 1 is the easiest of the five. You just need to remember to drink a tall glass of water right before each meal. Having your check-off chart on hand will remind you. Besides helping you eat less, the water will fix the mild-but-chronic dehydration problem that doctors say most Americans have.

When habits 2 and 3 are combined, the ratios get very interesting: you end up taking about the same time to eat a meal, but you enjoy it twice as much while consuming only half as much.

Habit 3 is the heart of this plan because it actually recalibrates your appetite. Remember, your appetite has the job of getting a certain amount of nourishment into your body. This can be achieved by eating a large quantity of poor-quality food or by eating a small quantity of high-quality food. If you exert your discipline and willpower by eating only half of whatever you normally eat, your appetite soon begins to realize that it can't get large quantities. Consequently, it gradually starts craving more quality instead of more quantity, and you begin to find nourishing food more and more appealing while junk food slowly and steadily seems less appealing.

Habits 4 and 5 are just plain hard, especially for the first few days. Because of habit 3, you will feel hungry between meals, and the fruit or vegetable of habit 4 will not be the most tempting snack. But as the days pass and your appetite adjusts from quantity to quality, these natural snacks will look better and better to you. And the saving grace of habit 5 is that exercise, while hard and sometimes boring, is also addictive, and the more consecutive days you do it, the more your body will appreciate the endorphins it releases.

What we discipline our bodies to do becomes a strong metaphor and guide for what we can also do with our minds and with our spirit.

Even as you begin to master the principles, the practices, and the habits of the physical Half Diet, you may start to understand that as beneficial and useful as this diet for the body is, there is a higher meaning, and what we discipline our bodies to do becomes a strong metaphor and guide for what we can also do with our minds and with our spirit.

The Half Diet is just beginning . . .

THE OTHER APPETITES

Most good performances have an intermission, and sometimes two of them: a time to get up, move around, ponder the first act, and get ready for the next one. You can talk and think very personally and candidly in an intermission and mentally prepare yourself for the next act. Books can have the same kind of break, and right now is a good moment for an intermission because, starting in the next chapter, we will begin to explore how the appetite for food is a "type" of all the other appetites that come with being human. In this intermission, I can help you see how the eat-half diet is a metaphor for how we can control all of our other appetites and for how we can strengthen our minds and our spirits as well as our bodies.

But before we get to that, let me mention a fortuitous or serendipitous thing that happened as I was writing this book. Just as I had finished Act I, about the physical Half Diet, I happened to be on an

> The eat-half diet is a metaphor for how we can control all of our other appetites and for how we can strengthen our minds and our spirits as well as our bodies.

airplane, and for want of anything better to do, I was reading *USA Today.* And there in black and white was the perfect study to back up the claims I had made.

PROOF FROM RHODE ISLAND

Proof shows up in the strangest places—there in my hands was an article by Nanci Hellmich titled "Study suggests eating slowly translates into eating less."[9] Here are some excerpts:

[In the study] . . . women [came] into a laboratory for lunch on two separate occasions. Each time, the women were offered a huge plate of pasta with tomato-vegetable sauce and grated Parmesan cheese, plus a glass of water. They were asked to eat until the point of comfortable fullness. On one occasion, they were instructed to eat as quickly as they could; on the other occasion they ate slowly and put down their spoons between bites.

They did not know the food and water [were] weighed before and after the meal to determine the amount consumed.

When eating quickly, the women consumed 646 calories in about nine minutes.

When eating more slowly, they had an average of 579 calories in about 29 minutes.

They ate 67 more calories in nine minutes than they did in 29 minutes," says lead researcher Kathleen Melanson, director of the [Rhode Island University] Energy Metabolism Laboratory. "If you add that up over three meals a day, that's a big difference in calories.

Upon completion of the meal and an hour afterward, the women were less satisfied and hungrier when eating quickly compared with then they ate slowly, she says. They said they enjoyed the meal more when they were taking their time.

Not surprisingly, the women drank more water when they

ate more slowly, and researchers are doing a follow-up study on whether that factor contributed to their feeling of fullness.

One way to help control calorie intake . . . "is to slow down and savor and enjoy your food more," Melanson says.

For the quick-eating test, volunteers used a large spoon, ate as quickly as possible, [and] didn't pause between bites. For the slow test, volunteers used a small spoon, took small bites, chewed food 15–20 times, [and] put the spoon down between bites."

So, there you go. It seems that the Half Diet has now been validated by a university's energy metabolism laboratory.

But any who have tried the Half Diet find that they don't need academic or research-based proof. Because the real proof lies in doing it ourselves. We feel better, we look better, and we end up eating better food and enjoying it more.

> But any who have tried the Half Diet find that they don't need academic or research-based proof. Because the real proof lies in doing it ourselves. We feel better, we look better, and we end up eating better food and enjoying it more.

MY HIDDEN AGENDA

As you have noticed, I was determined to stay with the "diet book" mentality for the first section of this book. However, you could probably tell that my tongue was partly in my cheek. What I really wanted to do was set up a model to talk about all appetites in general—which is my real interest and the real subject of this book.

That is not to say there was anything disingenuous or misleading about the physical diet I've proposed to you. It does work. It will work for anyone who implements it. Not only that, its results will make you more capable of

The physical, mental, and spiritual are not only connected, they are three parts of the same whole, and that whole is the soul.

understanding and implementing the mental diet and the spiritual diet that follow.

The physical, mental, and spiritual are not only connected, they are three parts of the same whole, and that whole is the soul. A physical body that is lean and clean, that is trim, strong, tuned, and hydrated, is infinitely better at receiving, conducting, and supporting the mental and spiritual processes that happen within. And that retuning can open up the whole universe to us.

We need to be sure we don't shortchange the reasons for and the ramifications of the physical diet, reducing our motives down to things such as a more attractive appearance or smaller dress size. Instead, let's elevate the idea of the physical diet to purposes such as longer life, clearer insights, and a purer intelligence and spirituality.

You have now read through the physical diet and decided (or are deciding whether or not) to do it. During this brief intermission, while you're thinking about it, let me add some other points, in the form of what I hope will be thought-prompting questions, for you to ponder. I've mentioned some of them briefly before, but these six questions will lead us into the mental and spiritual diets I have in mind and will begin to reveal where I'm really trying to take you in this book.

1. The God who made us could have used any means he wanted for us to "refuel" or to get the nutrients into our physical machines to keep them going (and growing). He could have designed it so we just tapped into a tree or a pond or some nutrient source through a tube or in some other utilitarian way, like gassing up a car. But instead, He made eating and drinking a pleasurable and infinitely varied experience and gave us appetites and tastes and expandable capacities. Why? Could it be that our food appetites are intentionally the physical representation of all our other appetites, and that

by learning to control that most obvious appetite, we can learn the principles that control all other appetites?

2. What if one of the most stunning ways in which man is different from animals is that animals manifest their destiny and fulfill their purpose by following and being subject to their instincts and appetites, while humans reach their fullest potential and gain their highest destiny by controlling and mastering their appetites? Perhaps our human qualities of patience and discipline, of the capacity to delay gratification and be proactive rather than reactive with regard to our appetites, are the very qualities that separate us most dramatically from the animals.

3. Why is it that the word "appetite" often carries a negative connotation unless it is modified by a positive adjective like "healthy"? By itself, it sounds a little like a foe or an enemy or at least an unpleasant challenge. But, in fact, isn't it appetites that make life exciting? They are our passions, the very drives and urges that motivate us and that make life enjoyable. Yes, they require controlling, but even that can be a pleasure. If we imagine a life without appetites, we find ourselves contemplating a flat, effortless, and boring state.

> Appetites make life exciting. If we imagine a life without appetites, we find ourselves contemplating a flat, effortless, and boring state.

4. Could joy be defined as appetite control? Is self-mastery ultimately the source, or at least the trigger, of our happiness?

5. Could there be not only a connection but also a wonderful sequence between body, mind, and spirit? Might these three provide related but separate and appropriately sequential ways of knowing and understanding things, with the sensory method leading

to the scientific method and finally being eclipsed by the spiritual method?

6.   In this larger perspective, might appetites be perceived as the passions and potential joys that come with this mortal opportunity, and could diets be viewed as how we choose to think and to live while we are here on earth?

EXPANDING OUR VIEW OF APPETITES

So what are our other appetites? Think for a minute before you turn the page and read on. Think about what you would put on the appetite list.

Without trying to be expansive or to sequence or categorize them in any particular way, here are some appetites:

- Recognition or acclaim
- Sex
- Sleep
- Ownership
- Control
- Independence
- Comfort
- Fame (or visibility or credit)
- Acceptance
- Achievement
- Position
- Ambition
- Power
- Wealth
- Love
- Understanding
- Knowledge
- Television and media
- Internet and technology
- Games and diversions

With the list in front of us (and it could be much longer), let's ask some key questions: What *are* appetites? Are they things we need? Things we want? Things we desire? Are they instincts? Natural attractions? Are they learned, or are they inherent?

For animals, appetites or instincts are built-in energy- and purpose-producing urges that allow them to survive. Are they more or less than that with us? Are we best served by subduing them or celebrating them?

Can we do both?

Here's a crack at defining an appetite: **something that *attracts* us but, if we let it, begins to *control* us and which, if unchecked, then becomes an *obsession* and, finally, if it is not mastered or bridled, turns into an addiction.**

With that definition in mind, what would you add to the appetite list?

Are there good and bad appetites? Are our longings for things such as love or wisdom too high and too pure to be called appetites? Are those with stronger or weaker appetites higher or lower beings?

Do any of these questions matter?

This book takes the view that these are the very questions that do matter—that they matter very much. Further, it takes the view that all appetites can be appreciated and understood and controlled by the same principles that work with our appetite for food.

> All appetites can be appreciated and understood and controlled by the same principles that work with our appetite for food.

The result of the physical diet is a body that is fit and strong and joyful. The result of the mental diet is a mind with the same characteristics. After the chapters devoted to the mental diet (ten of them, corresponding chapter by chapter with the ten chapters of the physical diet), we will need another intermission to set the stage for the final diet: the spiritual diet.

The physical diet and the loss of physical weight and the control of the appetite to eat are only the tip of the iceberg; the real challenge of human excellence is to master and control all of our appetites. Remember as you read that the appetite for food is a "type" or a metaphor for all of our other appetites, instincts, cravings, and desires. The principles that work for the physical also work for the emotional, mental, and spiritual constructs of life.

ACT II

THE MENTAL
HALF DIET

As you read on, compare the "physical"
chapters you have already read with the
upcoming "mental" chapters and note that
they take the same sequence and apply
the same principles.

Go back periodically to the corresponding physical topic, and use it as a comparison to better understand the mental/emotional chapters you are currently reading.

But as you move on and read on, keep working on and being committed to the physical diet! Work on it and try to get better and better at it because the physical diet will not only help you lose weight and become physically stronger, but it will also be the key by which you understand the deeper elements of fulfilling the measure of your creation by mastering and controlling the instincts and inclinations of your body, mind, and spirit (your whole soul)!

CHAPTER 11

"EAT HALF" MENTALLY

Compare to Chapter 1

I was climbing in the desert of southern Utah when I wrote this chapter, and I found myself at the mouth of a mysterious cave on the face of a red cliff. The cave was beautiful, with three huge white calla lilies blooming at its mouth and a high chimney at the back that revealed the bright blue sky through the opening far above. A cooing dove lived somewhere up in that rock chimney (you should have heard the echo of her call) and flew straight down to check on me every once in a while before flying straight back up again to her nest. I found the place so appealing that I sat, cross legged and guru-like, on a rock shelf at the opening of the cave and began to write.

The desert is a lot like the Half Diet. It is sparse. It is spare. It is beautiful, but not in an overly abundant or gluttonous way. At this time of year, it is all in bloom, with yellow flowers on the cacti and small, isolated blooms here

The desert is a lot like the Half Diet. It is sparse. It is spare. It is beautiful, but not in an overly abundant or gluttonous way.

and there in the sand. Because they are few and far between, you notice each blossom, each cactus, each individual flower separately, appreciating its unique, singular beauty, much like you enjoy food when you eat it one small, slow bite at a time. There is no junk here in the desert, no excess of vegetation, no stuff competing with other stuff.

SIMPLIFY

What power there is in simplification, in getting rid of excess, in focusing on one fine and worthwhile thing at a time! What a good mental diet it is to consume about half—to avoid all the excess that life puts in front of you, to keep your focus on the relatively few things that really matter, and to try to get rid of all the stuff that doesn't.

> Technology can fit the definition of appetite—first, it appeals; second, it begins to control us; third, it becomes an obsession; and fourth, it is an addiction.

Shut off your devices periodically. In fact, shut them off often. Don't even turn them on until you are ready to work or to answer texts or emails or social media. Put yourself in charge of when you turn on, log in, and go online, and don't do it any more often than you really choose. Remember how easily technology can fit the definition of appetite—first, it appeals; second, it begins to control us; third, it becomes an obsession; and fourth, it is an addiction. Stop the addiction while it is still in stage one!

And if you are already in stage two, three, or four, back it out, because there is no better way to simplify!

The demands of children can also be simplified. A woman I know was going nuts with the busyness and stress of her life. Her three boys had endless lessons or games or practices after school, sometimes two or three a night. She finally sat them down and said, "Boys, this is just too much. We never eat together, and we have no time to just relax and talk; something has to go. I have decided we will not do soccer next year." Instead of the cries of disappointment she had expected, the oldest boy smiled sheepishly and said, "Good, Mommy, because we really don't like soccer."

How many things in life are we doing just because everyone else is, or because we think we should, or because we want to keep up with the Joneses? Why do we let our lives become so overwhelming and so busy that we drive ourselves crazy doing things that may not really matter? As e. e. cummings said, "more / (& more & / still More) what the // hell are we all morticians?"[10]

The mental Half Diet is about simplifying and cutting out the excess busyness of our lives. It is about losing the "weight" of stress and fatigue.

A good way to start is by writing a personal mission statement that defines what is really important to you, then cutting out of your life the things that have nothing to do with your mission.

Another good way is to make a list of stewardship priorities each day:

- One meaningful, need-based thing you will do for someone in your family
- One meaningful, need-based thing you will do for someone at work or for a friend or acquaintance
- One meaningful, need-based thing you will do for yourself

These are the things that matter, and this is the mental diet that will help you lose the "pounds" of life's trivia and busyness that you don't want.

As you get more selective with your small screens, watch fewer big screens as well. Pick one or two TV shows that you really love and limit yourself to them. Use that excess TV time to take a walk or read a book or have a good conversation with someone you love.

Allow yourself a little solitude each day. Take a longer shower if that is the only place you are alone with your thoughts. Or go out in the garden and get your hands in the dirt. Or sit in a favorite chair and watch the sky.

Like the physical diet, the mental diet is not about trying to "eat" or juggle more things, but about being more selective and enjoying and taking time for the things that are truly good and that really matter. It's

Like the physical diet, the mental diet is not about trying to "eat" or juggle more things, but about being more selective and enjoying and taking time for the things that are truly good and that really matter.

about grabbing hold of your life and making thoughtful decisions about what you do, and about not just "eating" whatever is placed in front of you.

THE ADDICTIONS OF PERSONAL TECHNOLOGY

Play a guessing game with me. What am I thinking of that tastes good; that is "more-ish"; that is comfortable to do, especially when other things aren't going so well; that can be good and hearty, but is often damaging and unhealthy; that can be used as a pleasurable and sustaining asset, but that can also take over your life?

It could be food, right? That is the obvious answer, since the food appetite is the "type" for all other appetites. It could also be a lot of other things that appeal to our appetites. One thing it could be, and that it *is* for a lot of us: technology!—the personal and potentially addictive technologies of the Internet, laptops, email, video games, tablets, smartphones, GoPro cameras, downloads, Blackberrys, voicemail, PalmPilots, etc.

Think about the people you know (or are any of them you?) who can't sit through lunch without checking their texts or email or Instagram a couple of times, or their voicemail, or their social media pages; who only take their headphones off when they have to; who spend more time in virtual reality than in real reality; who sit down at their laptops and don't get up for hours; who text or talk on their cell phones while driving, shopping, eating, walking, working; who spend more time entering their to-do list than completing it; who feel anxiety attacks when they are out of wireless range or, heaven forbid, cell phone coverage.

For many, it is hard to imagine what they did with their time ten or fifteen years ago before personal electronic devices existed. More than half of their time is spent on them now, so what did they do with that half of their time back then? Maybe they read books, or did sports, or walked, or went out in nature, or attended the theater, or visited, in person, with other human beings. Imagine that!

The questions we should ask ourselves are so similar to the questions an overeating person has to ask himself. What could you do if you weren't eating (or surfing the Internet or using social media or playing video games) all the time? What would you feel like if you were not carrying all that extra weight (extra useless information)? What is all that food (data) doing to you, to your outlook, your brain, your body? Why is the bad food (bad sites, games, etc.) the most addictive of all?

The cures would be similar, too: take smaller portions, consume only at certain times of the day, turn off the technology and ignore it at other times, maybe cut your time-use of it in half, and see if your brain starts wanting better stuff from technology when you only consume half as much—see if you start wanting more quality as you restrict your quantity.

Is technology bad? Do our personal electronic devices have to take over our lives? Of course not—just as food is not bad and eating does not have to take over our lives. But as with any appetite, there can be that dangerous, even insidious progression from appetite to obsession to addiction.

It is so important to think of technology as a tool, as a means to other desired ends, and not as an end in itself. Just as with food, if we limit our intake by confining our use to certain restricted times of the day, it will become necessary to use that limited time more effectively. We will go only to the sites that really help us, make only the calls we need to make, and listen only to the music that really uplifts.

A good way to check yourself (and to check your appetite for technology) is to simply ask yourself, fairly often, the old question we asked about the food appetite: "Who's winning? Who is in charge here—me or the technology?" If your smartphone is always on and you feel you have to answer it every time it rings, or at least see who it is, or check Facebook every ten minutes, or look at each notification immediately, then your device is winning. If those white headphone cords are always connected to your ears, you are obsessed. If you spend more time on video games than on exercising, or on personal planning, or on reading scriptures or attending church, you might be more addicted than you think.

Learn to *use* the marvels of technology to help you reach conscious goals. Think of electronic devices as *tools* that can help you to be what you want to be and accomplish what you want to do. But be in charge. Think it through. Use technology according to your rules and priorities, and don't let it pull you into someone else's idea of what is interesting or important.

CHAPTER 12

WHAT LIVING LIFE AT HALF SPEED WILL DO FOR YOU

Compare to Chapter 2

The laws that govern our food intake can be extended to other areas of our lives. In many instances, our spiritual lives can be mirrored in our physical situations. Laws that govern the physical can also govern the mental.

The promise of the physical diet (recall from Chapter 2) was (and is) that as you cut the quantity intake of food by half, your body will start desiring and demanding better quality from what you do put in your mouth. If you seek out quality nutrients, junk and fast food will soon begin to look less appetizing and vegetables and fruit will look better and better.

The same principle works with your mind. As you cut some of the trash and non-nourishing stuff out of your life, as you simplify, your soul will gradually begin to appreciate and even crave more quality in your activities, your entertainment, your interests, and your relationships.

As you cut some of the trash and non-nourishing stuff out of your life, as you simplify, your soul will gradually begin to appreciate and even crave more quality.

Consider how you use your time and what appeals to you. If you are overloaded, it becomes harder to enjoy the high-quality activities. Museums will never be very appealing if you spend all your time at amusement parks. Art galleries won't attract you if all you see is video games. The symphony or ballet will not beckon if you only go to comic book–based movies.

In the physical diet, the key to eating half as much is to eat twice as slowly. Slow down the way you eat—smaller bites, more chewing, savoring each morsel. When you do this, your body rewards you by enjoying food more, craving quality, and getting fitter and stronger. In life, we need to do the same thing with our time and mind. As you slow down and simplify the way you live and the way you think, your brain rewards you by producing better ideas and purer thoughts, by noticing more beauty, by becoming more perceptive and more aware.

In our world today, the pace of life has become so fast. We rush from one thing to the next without taking time to notice or even to think. Some of us remember slower times when evenings were long enough to sit and talk and even have dinner together. Kids had time to just play and create, weekends were a time to relax and recharge, and summer had some lazy, hazy days.

As you slow down and simplify the way you live and the way you think, your brain rewards you by producing better ideas and purer thoughts.

Today, the average fast food meal takes six minutes to consume, our evenings are busier than our days, our kids are as overscheduled as we are, and we have developed what Guy

Claxton, a British psychologist, calls "an inner psychology of speed, of saving time and maximizing efficiency." Everything seems to be geared toward getting more done in less time.

SLOWING DOWN

Carl Honoré, in his book *In Praise of Slow*, puts much of modern life in perspective when he honors speed but also worries about it:

> Speed has helped to remake our world in ways that are wonderful and liberating. Who wants to live without the Internet or jet travel? The problem is that our love of speed, our obsession with doing more and more in less and less time, has gone too far; it has turned into an addiction, a kind of idolatry.
>
> Even when speed starts to backfire, we invoke the go-faster gospel. Falling behind at work? Get a quicker Internet connection. No time for that novel you got at Christmas? Learn to speed-read. Diet not working? Try liposuction. Too busy to cook? Buy a microwave.
>
> And yet some things cannot, should not, be sped up. They take time; they need slowness. When you accelerate things that should not be accelerated, when you forget how to slow down, there is a price to pay.[11]

One London-based life coach quoted in Honoré's book puts it this way: "Burnout used to be something you mainly found in people over forty. Now I'm seeing men and women in their thirties, and even in their twenties, who are completely burned out."[12] Perhaps we would do well to remember what Gandhi said: "There is more to life than increasing its speed."

Even our kids, who used to have both time and spontaneity, are now overprogrammed. A recent cartoon said it all: Two little girls are standing at the school bus stop, each clutching a smartphone with a calendar app. One says to the other, "OK, I'll move ballet back an hour, reschedule gymnastics, and cancel piano. You shift your violin lesson to Thursday and skip soccer practice. That gives us from 3:15 to 3:45 on Wednesday the 16th to play."[13]

Another cartoon, this one by Tom Cheney in the *New Yorker*, shows two primary school boys walking down a street, books under their arms, baseball caps on their heads. With a world-weariness beyond their years, one mutters to the other: "So many toys—so little unstructured time."

The culture of hurry gets even more intense for college students. The stress of trying to do everything and do it all fast got so intense at Harvard that the dean of the undergraduate school, Harry Lewis, wrote an open letter that now goes out to every first-year Harvard student. The title of the letter is *Slow Down*.

The old saying "haste makes waste" is true. Hurrying all the time not only makes us botch things, but it also wastes our peace and wrests the quality from our lives.

During the course of seven pages, Lewis makes the case for getting more out of university—and life—by doing less. He urges students to "think twice about racing through their degrees and to avoid piling on too many extracurricular activities. Do fewer things and take the time to make the most of them," he says, "and remember that doing nothing at times, and slowing yourself down, is an essential part of good thinking."

"Empty time is not a vacuum to be filled," writes the dean. "It is the thing that enables the other things on your mind to be creatively rearranged, like the empty square in the 4x4 puzzle that makes it possible to move the other fifteen pieces around."[14]

One lesson of the New Testament story of Mary and Martha may never have been more relevant than it is now. We find ourselves like Jesus described Martha, "cumbered about"[15] and "careful and troubled about many things,"[16] trying to do everything for everyone and missing what really matters. We find ourselves unable to be like Mary, who "[chose] the better part."[17]

What we need to do is consciously slow down. Slowing down physically can help us slow down mentally. Make yourself walk a little slower and notice a little more, drive a little slower and be more aware of what is around you. You will lose only a few seconds, and you will start to win the battle against haste and hurry. The old saying "haste makes waste" is true. Hurrying all the time not only makes us botch things, but it also wastes our peace and wrests the quality from our lives. How many times a day do we say "hurry" to our kids (or to ourselves)?

CALMING DOWN

Find the things that calm you, slow your mind down. For some, it is gardening. For one man I know, it is archery—the solitude of shooting arrows at a target. For many, classical music soothes and slows of their souls.

We said earlier that everything seems to be geared toward getting more done in less time. Well, think for a minute about all of your various appetites as interlocking gears, some bigger, some smaller, that turn together. Appetites for food, for success, for recognition, for wealth, for sex, for control, for status—all are gears turning.

What is the "drive gear," the one that powers all the others? Perhaps it is the appetite for hurry, for haste, for speed. We want everything faster. We overload our lives and think the way to get everything done is to hurry more. That sense of pace feeds each of our appetites and causes all of them pull harder on us.

If we can slow down some of those interlocking gears, they all begin to slow down and we begin to resist the drive gear of hurry and haste. Our hunger for food, the appetite that serves as such a good metaphor for all the others, is a good place to start. By sipping and savoring small bites and eating half, we change the unhealthy rush of quick-quantity refueling to a pleasurable tasting of quality food. And the very process of slowing down that gear begins to slow down the others. We taste, and as we are tasting, we start seeing more and hearing more, and thinking more.

If you can slow down eating, you start to feel that you can slow down other things. Let that kiss for your loved one linger a little longer. Look into a person's eyes and hold their hand a half second longer when you greet them. Sit down and take a look around you for a moment before you start a job at work.

Fast thinking, the kind of thinking we do under pressure (when the clock is ticking), often produces tunnel vision and reduces our awareness of the things around us. Slow thinking is intuitive and creative. Slowing down and giving ideas time to simmer at their own pace yields rich and subtle insights. It leads to lateral thinking and creativity and serendipity.

Plato believed that the highest form of leisure was to be still and receptive to the world. Franz Kafka put it this way: "You do not need to leave your room. Remain sitting at your table and listen. Do not even listen; simply wait. Do not even wait. Be quite still and solitary. The world will freely offer itself to you to be unmasked. It has no choice. It will roll in ecstasy at your feet."

> Fast thinking, the kind of thinking we do under pressure (when the clock is ticking), often produces tunnel vision and reduces our awareness of the things around us. Slow thinking is intuitive and creative.

As your mind slows down and calms down, you begin to discover something that is hard to explain logically but wonderful to feel. It is "the speed of going slow." Though it seems counterintuitive and incongruent, as you slow down and become more peaceful and aware, you actually get where you are going or finish what you need to do more easily and, somehow, more quickly. The lights turn green for you, the people you need answer their phones or your texts, and life takes on a more pleasant rhythm. Rudyard Kipling wrote of keeping your head while all about you are losing theirs.[18] Today, we need to learn to keep our cool while all around us are losing theirs, and to stay slow inside even as we work to meet a deadline or to get the children to school on time.

The speed of going slow is not something you learn overnight or something that works all the time. But it is something you can learn and something you can practice. Eat slowly, walk slowly, think slowly, try for more awareness and perspective, taste more, see more, feel more, and look for more quality and less quantity in your activities, your relationships, and your goals as well as in your food.

> The speed of going slow is not something you learn overnight or something that works all the time. But it is something you can learn and something you can practice.

CHAPTER 13

SIPPING, SAVORING, AND SMELLING YOUR LIFE

Compare to Chapter 3

When our food appetite controls us, we rush through meals, gorging ourselves, animal-like, and missing much of the taste and enjoyment. When our other appetites, lusts, and instincts control us (particularly the pervasive appetite for hurry and haste), we rush through our days, missing much of the beauty and subtlety that makes life worth living.

On the other hand, when we control our food appetite—sipping, savoring, and smelling our food rather than gorging, gulping, and guzzling it—we can appreciate and taste every morsel. When we control our other appetites (for work, for control, for instant gratification, and especially for haste), we begin to find the moments of joy that are the very purpose of life.

When we control our other appetites (for work, for control, for instant gratification, and especially for haste), we begin to find the moments of joy that are the very purpose of life.

The last chapter focused on doing things more slowly to gain more awareness. Now think about it in reverse. Can being more aware enable us to slow down?

Stress-producing haste and impatience often come from a habitual focus on the future. We are thinking about where we need to be and what we need to do, and with our mind out there in front, we pull ourselves headlong through the present, not even noticing the beauty, the people, and the opportunities slipping past us.

Telling (and willing) ourselves to slow down (Chapter 12) is important, but the other half of the formula is to increase our observational powers and our awareness of what is around us—to live more in the present and appreciate the moment we are in. Those who learn to do this receive many rewards:

- Enjoyment of both the sensual and the spiritual beauty that is always around them
- Serendipitous acquaintances, opportunities, ideas, and even short-cuts to where they are trying to go
- A slower, less stressed attitude that makes them somehow more efficient (the speed of going slow)

Of course, we need to think ahead, to plan, to make our lists. But once they are made, we need to learn to shift back into the present and notice and enjoy all that is here. After all, the present is the only place we ever actually live!

AWARENESS AS THE SLOWING AGENT

Some people can induce an inner calm simply by commanding themselves to slow down (eating more slowly, walking more slowly, etc., as discussed in the last chapter). Others, like a horse straining at the bit, just become jumpier and more anxious when forced to go slower.

The key for this second type of person is to focus on awareness instead of on slowing down. Do what you need to do: run your errands, check off your list, make your calls, feed the family, get the kids ready, do your work—but while you are doing it, tune in to the present that is all around you. Be aware of smells and sounds. Notice and appreciate things as well as just seeing them. Feel textures, smell aromas, and really taste what you eat. In other words, sip, savor, and smell your life rather than guzzling, gulping, and gorging it.

The reason the Half-Diet Diet works is that as we eat less and eat more slowly (reducing quantity), we enjoy more (increase quality) and are motivated to continue the pattern. As we become better and better at enjoying more—at sipping and savoring—we find it easier and easier to eat more slowly and to eat less.

> Tune in to the present that is all around you. Be aware of smells and sounds. Notice and appreciate things. In other words, sip, savor, and smell your life rather than guzzling, gulping, and gorging it.

It is a classic chicken-and-egg situation. Whether you start with the "egg" of slowing down or with the "chicken" of enjoying more, one will lead to the other, and you will have both. With all appetites, slowing down increases awareness and enjoyment, and increasing awareness and enjoyment causes a slowing down.

With eating, the first bite or two is easy to enjoy because you are hungry and the food tastes good. But as you shovel the rest of the meal in, satisfying the appetite, the joy-per-bite quotient drops. It takes awareness and conscious decisions to sip and savor to keep the enjoyment level up.

"First bites" in life are also easy to enjoy—the first time in a new place, the first ski run of the morning after a snowstorm, the first day of school or a new job. But when routine and the pressure to get everything done set in, we find ourselves riding the lift one more time just to get our money's worth or mechanically plowing through the day rather than enjoying it. We rush around without awareness, satisfying our appetite to get things done but not enjoying much of it along the way. Through deliberate, conscious awareness, we begin to notice things that bring back the joy and slow down the tyranny of time.

> See your awareness as an antidote to your appetites. Let your senses sharpen and slow you down and bring you peace.

Our senses are intended to be the receptors of joy. The better we use them and tune them, the more we receive.

I once met a blind man in the busy center of a city, sitting quietly on a street corner with his dog, selling baskets he had made. As I spoke with him, he must have detected pity in my tone, and he didn't like it. Politely but firmly, he told me that while I had one sense (sight) that was better than his, he had four that were better than mine. He then proceeded to tell me of sounds he could hear that I could not, and smells, and things he could feel and taste, even there in the clamor of the city. He even told me some things about myself that I don't know to this day how he perceived. His joy came from his awareness, not from rushing around doing things.

Learn to sip and savor your life, to appreciate new perspectives, to relish the beauty and intrigue of the present, to fine-tune your senses, to live in the moment. See your awareness as an antidote to your appetites. Let your senses sharpen and slow you down and bring you peace.

CHAPTER 14

THE PURE WATER OF CLEAR THOUGHT AS YOUR KEY ALLY

Compare to Chapter 4

As I sit down to write this morning, I have my favorite water bottle sitting on the table beside my keyboard. I will sip away at it, and by the time I finish this chapter, I will likely have finished the one liter it holds and be halfway to my daily goal of drinking two liters of water. Full hydration is a big part of the Half-Diet Diet. This pure, clear H_2O is what cleanses and lubricates and refreshes the body. I take this favorite bottle pretty much everywhere I go. It's in the cup holder when I am driving and on my desk when I'm at work. If I'm a little behind on my water consumption, I even take it in the shower with me. It makes the two-liter-a-day goal easy. I've also started drinking three tall glasses of water in the bathroom each morning as I take my fish oil and vitamin pills. Getting that much water into myself early somehow makes the whole day ahead look easier.

Back in Chapter 4, we advocated making water your ally by getting in the habit of drinking a full glass of water before each meal. A stomach full of water doesn't have room for too much food. Chapter 4 went on to say:

Drinking a full glass before eating results in two good things:
- More water (which your body needs)
- Less food (which your body doesn't need)

Both are accomplished by the simple resolution that becomes a habit: "Before I eat anything—meals or snacks—I will drink a glass of water." Filling your stomach partway up with water is the simplest conceivable way to make less room in there for food. And staying fully hydrated (something very few of us do consistently) makes you feel better in all sorts of ways.

The same principle and habit works in the mental diet, but the clear water is replaced by clear thought and the habit we need to develop is to always drink in some of that pure thought before we jump into eating away at any kind of action.

DON'T JUST DO SOMETHING; SIT THERE!

Scripture tells us that God created all things spiritually before he made them physically.[19] What a lesson. Think things through before trying to do them. Take the time to plan. Sharpen your saw before you try to cut with it.

> Take the time to plan. Sharpen your saw before you try to cut with it. Think a minute about *why* you are doing something as well as *how* you are going to do it.

Think a minute about *why* you are doing something as well as *how* you are going to do it.

People who are chronically dehydrated (and a high percentage of us are) are people who get out of the habit of drinking water. And people who are in chronic ruts or routines are people who have gotten out of the habit of thinking. The days just go by, one blurring into the next, and we end up doing the same things, putting out the same fires, following the same schedules, until we are almost doing things in our sleep. Thought can change it; a new idea, a new perspective, a new way to do something can wake us up and hydrate our minds.

Challenge yourself a little. Ask, "Is this really what I want to do? Is this really the way I want to do it?" Or, if you want to challenge yourself a little more, ask, "Is this really what God wants me to do? Is this really the way He wants me to do it?"

What appetite are we overcoming here? On the physical level, the water helps curb and control our appetite for food. On the mental level, more conscious thought helps us to master our appetite for constant action and activity. Action is an addiction in today's world. "Don't just sit there; do something!"

Instead, most of us need the opposite advice: "Don't just do something; sit there!"

> Action is an addiction in today's world. "Don't just sit there; do something!"
>
> Instead, most of us need the opposite advice: "Don't just do something; sit there!"

Sit there for a moment and think. Don't just do something to be busy or to be active. Do things because you have thought about them and decided to do them, and how to do them, and why you are doing them. We live in a world of frenetic and often frantic activity, and we have been almost conned into thinking that resting, waiting, pausing, and thinking are forms of laziness. As with food, the goal is not more quantity but more quality in the things we choose to do and in how we do them.

SHARPEN YOUR SAW

The best kind of thought is the unhurried, peaceful, creative thought in which you ask yourself questions and let answers come. The kind of hurried, pressure-packed thinking we do sometimes—such as cramming for a test or preparing at the last moment for a meeting or an assignment—is kind of like stuffing yourself when you are hungry. Slower, more aware, and more sensitive thinking is what we are trying to achieve with the Half-Diet Diet.

Three stories come to mind:

One summer, our family was working together on building a summer cabin. We were not experienced builders, but we had plans and tools and instruction books and thought we could do it. We kept making small mistakes because we were rushing into things, anxious to get it built and be finished. The mistakes were making things take twice as long, and we finally realized that the thinking was more important than the doing, and that five minutes of thought often revealed a better way or gave us a warning about some pitfall we were about to tumble into. We developed a simple motto that saved us: "Think three times, measure twice, and build once." It applies to almost every aspect of life.

We spend our vacation time each summer in a very rural farming area, and one of the goals is to relax and slow down and think. One of the interesting side benefits of this attitude is that I can do things there that I never thought I could do—and that I haven't been able to do anywhere else. The hydraulics on the tractor died one summer, and, since I was in the thought mode, I just sat there and looked at it for a half hour or so. I traced the lines with my eyes, seeing what went from where and trying to understand how the system worked. To my great surprise, I began to understand hydraulic systems just by observing, and I discovered the problem and fixed it myself. I had a similar experience with a sprinkler system and another one with a boat engine. I, who had never fixed anything in my life, fixed some fairly complex things just by thinking!

The last story is from my childhood. As a small boy, I lived near my Swedish grandfather, who occasionally took me to the woodworking shop at the university where he taught cabinetry just to let me hammer or saw a bit. One day (I must have been about eight), he handed me a crosscut saw and a two-by-four and invited me to saw off a piece. I sawed with vigor, but very little happened. The tiny cut in the board hardly deepened, and when I sawed harder, the cut started turning black as though I were trying to burn through it rather than saw through it. Waiting until my frustration peaked, my grandfather took the saw and, quickly and efficiently, with a little file, sharpened it.

When he handed it back to me, it was like a miracle. As I drew it back and pushed it forward, it chewed through the board. Even the sound it made was fulfilling. *Vroom, vroom.* Before I knew it, the saw was through and the severed part of the board dropped to the floor. "Before you work," Grandfather said, "sharpen your saw."

> "Before you work," Grandfather said, "sharpen your saw."

Remember, as with the water before the meal, it is the sequence that matters. Drinking a glass of water after eating does not do as much good as drinking it before, and thinking about how and why to do something after you did it doesn't do as much good as thinking it through beforehand. And keep in mind that fleeting thoughts do not do as much good as captured thoughts. Like carrying a water bottle around to remind yourself to drink, carry a notepad or little pocket booklet and pen around or have a note-taking app on your phone. Jot down thoughts as you have them. Sit there for a minute and let a thought or an idea develop, then capture it in writing.

EXERCISING THE MIND

Compare to Chapter 5

Back in Chapter 5, we discussed the importance of finding a form of physical exercise that you love and challenged you to engage in that lovable form of fitness at least five times per fortnight. Though it is not directly about food or the appetite for food, exercise is a legitimate part of a physical diet because it uses the food. The food is the input, and the exercise is the output.

Exercise puts the fuel we take in to the good use of building muscle and skill and heart/lung capacity and does not leave fuel for the bad use of adding weight or accumulating fat. In a successful diet, the appetite for output

Just as physical exercise tones and trims the body and keeps excess weight off, so mental exercise tones and trims the mind and holds at bay the dimming and dulling that can come to an idle or passive mind.

(exercise) balances and harmonizes the appetite for input (food) and both appetites, held in check by each other, work to our benefit.

We all know that the mind needs exercise, too, and just as physical exercise tones and trims the body and keeps off excess weight, so mental exercise tones and trims the mind and holds at bay the dimming and dulling that can come to an idle or passive mind.

Just as with food, it is about cultivating and controlling an input appetite and an output appetite and balancing the two of them. Mentally, the input appetite is for awareness, stimulation, information, knowledge, data, understanding, etc. and the output appetite is for accomplishing something or contributing something or impressing someone by turning those inputs into outputs.

On the one side, we should learn to control what kind of inputs we let in. We can monitor ourselves to take into our minds quality rather than junk. On the other side, we should strive not only to keep our minds active and fit but also to control how and to what ends we use our minds and their amazing capacity.

Once again, the physical is truly a "type" for the mental.

Just as we expand muscle and extend our skill and capacity by working out physically, so we enhance our mental faculties by working out our minds. A person who has a physically active job may need less additional exercise, and a constantly intellectually challenged student or someone who is constantly stimulated and mentally tested in her job may need less outside or additional mental exercise.

And just as we must find physical exercise that we enjoy if it is to become a consistent and pleasurable habit, so we must engage in types of mental stimulation that we enjoy if they are to become something we gravitate to and do out of love more than out of duty. Crossword or Sudoku puzzles may be pleasurable mental exercises for one, mathematic problems for another, writing historical fiction for one, attending discussion groups for another. We must each find our own combination.

INPUT VS. OUTPUT

But remember that we are talking about output here, not input. It is important to separate the two. The input of reading or studying or listening to music is like eating, so to say "Reading is my mental exercise" is a little like saying "Eating is my physical exercise." Reading is often our input, and the higher the quality of the material, the better, but it is what we do with the learning or perceptions we gain that forms our output.

In the physical diet, we are trying to decrease the quantity and increase the quality of what we eat while simultaneously expanding what our bodies can do with good, enjoyable exercise and the nourishment that our disciplined eating brings in. In the mental diet, we are trying to get rid of mental junk food and bring in wholesome, clear thought, and then use that mental nourishment to apply our minds to work and creativity that we love and that matters.

> Find a form of output mental exercise (creating or solving something) that you love, and engage in it at least a couple of times a week.

So the mental challenge is similar to the physical one. Find a form of output mental exercise (creating or solving something) that you love, and engage in it at least a couple of times a week (or five times per fortnight). Let your own desires, appetites, and likes be your guide. It might be writing poetry or fiction. It might be painting or drawing. It might be logic problems or jigsaw puzzles. It might be songwriting or music performance. If all else fails, or if you just love tests and puzzles and mental problems to solve, check out one of the many memory-strengthening, Alzheimer's-fighting mental puzzle sites that have cropped up all over the Internet. The best mental exercise creates or solves even as it makes your mind work.

CHAPTER 16

MENTAL FASTING (AND SLOWING)

Compare to Chapter 6

'm sure the chapter on fasting as part of the physical diet (Chapter 6) was no surprise to most readers. The physical and dietary benefits of fasting are well established. Applying the same principle to the mind may be a bit trickier.

But let's start by thinking back to Chapter 6 (physical fasting) for a minute. What that chapter said, in essence, was that fasting cleanses the body and increases awareness. Remember that everything physical, particularly when it comes to appetite and dieting, is a "type" or a teaching symbol for a mental or spiritual truth.

Physically, we fast by not taking nourishment for a period. What is the mental equivalent? We know that both the body and the mind have need for nourishment. The body is nourished by the intake of food, and the mind is nourished by the intake of information, ideas, and insights. Fasting, both physical and mental, is about halting our intake and cutting off our external nourishment for a period so we can turn more within

> There are not too many thoughts or too many ideas—just too much junk thought and too many bad ideas, and we occasionally need to clean house mentally.

ourselves and be more in touch with our soul and our spirit.

At this point, you might say, "Wait a minute; you're comparing physical food to mental thought and knowledge and education? And you're saying we should fast from thinking? Why would I want to not think? I know I eat too much food, but is there such a thing as too much thought?"

Think about it for a minute (excuse the pun). We don't fast because there is too much food but because there is too much junk food, and because our systems need to shut down and rest occasionally. Fasting cleans us out and resets and recommits us to better quality. Similarly, there are not too many thoughts or too many ideas—just too much junk thought and too many bad ideas, and we occasionally need to clean house mentally. By trying not to think for a period—trying to close out all the noisy clamor of the world—we reset our minds toward quality thought and begin to discover the treasures within.

When we are eating, our body has to be busy chewing and digesting and replenishing our systems. Physical fasting is turning off the intake so everything can rest and refresh and restart. When we are inputting data and stimuli and concepts, our mind has to be busy processing and analyzing and remembering them. Mental fasting is to discontinue the intake for a while and let the mind reboot and respond to what is going on inside of it.

MEDITATION

So you have probably guessed it by now: mental fasting is meditation. And what is meditation? It is just what we have been saying—shutting off the outside stimulus and turning off the normal mental pattern so the brain can stop digesting for a while and just be still and peaceful and rediscover itself.

There are many meditation techniques, and most of them make meditation sound and feel much more complicated than it has to be. Meditation, best defined, is simply mental fasting—turning off the usual "digestion" of analyzing, concentrating, calculating, and processing information and putting the mind at rest.

You can meditate with a mantra, a sound like *ommm* that you repeat and focus on. You can meditate by breathing deeply and trying to think only about the air going in and out of your lungs. You can meditate with the Zen technique of just sitting, quiet and relaxed, and emptying your mind. But let me tell you my favorite way to meditate. It has only three steps:

> Mental fasting is meditation—shutting off the outside stimulus and turning off the normal mental pattern so the brain can stop digesting for a while and just be still and peaceful and rediscover itself.

1. Sit in a comfortable spot and relax. If there is a lot of tension in you, relax your body one part at a time: first your head and neck, then your shoulders, and so on.

2. Remind yourself that you exist in the here and now. You are in the present. It has never been this moment before and you have never been exactly here before, so everything is new.

3. Be aware of everything around you and in you. Don't concentrate on anything or analyze anything or try to figure anything out. Just be aware. Be aware of what is inside your body: your breath, your heart beating, your kidneys filtering your blood, your hair and nails growing slowly, your skin reproducing and replacing its cells. Be aware of everything outside of you: the temperature,

> The physical fasting challenge is one day a month. Since the mind is much, much faster than the body, mental fasting ought to happen more often. Find a little time to meditate every day, even if just for a couple of minutes.

the atmospheric pressure, sounds, smells, how the air feels on your skin. Accept everything as it is and simply be aware of it. Use your whole mind for awareness. Don't let it go off on tangents or worries or conclusions. Just be aware.

The physical fasting challenge is one day a month. Since the mind is much, much faster than the body, mental fasting ought to happen more often. Find a little time to meditate every day, even if just for a couple of minutes, and find more time on Sundays when you can sit for a while and really become comfortable with meditation—when you can be still and know.

There is much more to say on this subject, but I must save some of it for Act III, the spiritual diet. Keep in mind that we are still in Act II, the mental diet, and that there will be a corresponding spiritual chapter later. In the meantime, learn and enjoy the art of mental fasting, which the world calls "meditation."

CHAPTER 17

GIVING BACK (AND KNOWING WHEN YOU HAVE ENOUGH)

Compare to Chapter 7

I f you recall, Chapter 7 was a major departure, because with it, the physical diet ceased to be about just you! If you think back to that chapter, the physical diet suddenly became very different from any and all other diets because it was not only about you losing weight—it was also about the needs of other people.

Chapter 7 told you that just eating half was not enough—that it was important to give the half you didn't eat to someone who needed it. And it suggested some simple, inexpensive ways to sponsor a third-world child or assist in feeding the homeless. At that point, the physical diet was about doing the right thing as well as doing the smart thing. It was about helping others as well as helping yourself. It was about other people's need to eat more as well as about your need to eat less.

Stated another way: One reason to eat less is that you don't need that much food and your body is better off without it. The other reason not to eat so much is that other people are starving and the half you don't eat can feed someone else.

It's the same with all appetites. One reason for controlling them is that you are better off if you do. The other reason is that others can be better off if you consume less—less money, less material, less fossil fuel, less of anything that you don't really need.

> One reason for controlling them is that you are better off if you do. The other reason is that others can be better off if you consume less—less money, less material, less fossil fuel, less of anything that you don't really need.

Can you feed the world or eradicate hunger by eating less? No. But can you help other individuals by giving away your excess and, in the process, feel better about others and about the world and about yourself? Yes.

Can you stop global warming or stop poverty or improve the self-image of the universe by consuming less? No. But can you improve the world just a bit and make it a little better place for other people by using less and acquiring less and controlling your appetites for everything from material wealth to sex? Yes.

Appetites are all about consumption. In the New Testament, James warns against wanting things for the wrong reason: "that ye may consume it upon your lusts."[20] A "lust" is often nothing more than an uncontrolled appetite. When we want things and consume things simply to satisfy our lusts, we have made a serious error involving a spiritual confusion between means and ends.

If hunger or appetite or lust controls us, then eating or obtaining or controlling or getting things becomes an end in itself and is often destructive both to others and to ourselves. But when we control our appetite, food is the means to other ends. It gives us the energy to do good and to fulfill our stewardships.

It is the same with all appetites. If we seek wealth as a means to help others and bring about good works, we are in control of that appetite. Likewise, we can view our appetite for sex as the means to the end of showing our love and commitment to our spouse.

> We need to understand the concept of "enough," that *things* should only be the means to more worthy ends and that giving what we do not need to others is the key to *our* joy as well as theirs.

Viewing controlled appetites as the means to good and worthy ends causes us to make good decisions and to appreciate the energy and motivation that appetites give us. And there is pleasure and joy in the means! Everyone knows the old cliché about happiness being a journey rather than a destination. Appetites, viewed as the means, become joyful and lead to worthy ends.

Again, the bridle metaphor: The horse is not the end but the means—not the destination but the method of getting there. But what joy there is in riding him (so long as he is in our control, so long as he is bridled)! Slow your appetites, bring them into control, make them work for your efforts to give and to serve. Then you will be filled with love.

THREE OTHER APPETITES

The appetite for food is the perfect "type" for other appetites. We control our food appetite, eat less, and give more. Look at three other appetites as parallels:

1. *The appetite for wealth or accumulation.* So often, uncontrolled, this appetite involves all taking and no giving. We say, "All I want

is the land next to mine." And it never stops. We want more and more. What we have is never enough. I repeat e. e. cummings's observation: " more / (& more & / still More) what the // hell are we all morticians?" Understanding the physical diet teaches us that more is not always better, that less is often more. We need to understand the concept of "enough," that *things* should only be the means to more worthy ends and that giving what we do not need to others is the key to *our* joy as well as theirs.

2. *The appetite for sex.* Do we consume this appetite on our own lusts? Do we think too much about our own needs and pleasure and not enough about our spouse's? Can thinking more about giving make sex the means to the end of showing deeper and truer love? If so, it may affect the names we use for intimacy. "Making love" implies the creation of additional feeling for an exclusive other, while "having sex" sounds like scratching an itch or satisfying an appetite.

> "Making love" implies the creation of additional feeling for an exclusive other, while "having sex" sounds like scratching an itch or satisfying an appetite.

3. *The appetite for independence.* What a lust this is! We want financial independence, emotional independence, social independence. We get duped into thinking that needing others is a weakness. In fact, what we have, and what we should want, is *interdependence*. The world functions on financial interdependence—giving and receiving—and our emotional and social life are the same. The more we focus on the giving, and on needs rather than wants, the more we control this appetite and the more joy we find. Self-reliance can be good, but only when it is the means to being useful to others and to the world.

In this concept lies a good definition for the controlling of appetites. Control is first. Consuming less and less is second. Giving what you do not consume is the third part of the definition. It adds up to a classic win-win situation in which you help yourself by helping others. It works on the micro as well as the macro level. If you fast and donate the money you saved by not eating, that money helps others and everyone wins. If this country finds ways to conserve energy, we are better off and so are other countries that need more. If you take your somewhat spoiled and somewhat unappreciative children on a humanitarian expedition to a third-world village to help dig a well or build a clinic, you save lives over there, and you just may save your own child's emotional life as he begins to become aware of his blessings and of his abilities to give and to serve.

CHAPTER 18

THE POETIC PART

Compare to Chapter 8

What in the world is a *"poetic diet"*? That was the question many readers asked as they started Chapter 8, before the explanation and the guarantee that writing poetry would help them lose weight. Specifically, Chapter 8—back when we were still dealing with only the physical diet—said that being aware of the quality and amount of what you eat . . . appreciating it . . . tasting it . . . sipping and savoring it . . . has a lot to do with our ability to be aware and sensitive in the broader and more general sense, and writing poetry, or trying to, is a great way to improve awareness and sensitivity.

In other words, there is a connection between our perception, our perspective, and our self-discipline. A glutton is not very aware or perceptive. His attention is taken up by fulfilling his appetite. He eats quickly. His appetite is controlling him. One who "sips and savors" takes control of his appetite, "bridles it," if you will, reining it in and using it, at the pace he dictates, for his pleasure and enjoyment. Quality takes over for quantity.

The important thing to realize is that the connection between awareness and appetite control works both ways. When we eat more slowly and bridle the appetite for food, we become more aware of the taste, texture, and enjoyment of our small, slow bites. And working on awareness and poetic sensitivity slows us down and removes the gluttony. It is the same with all appetites: as we control them and slow them down, we begin to notice more and to appreciate more. And as we train ourselves to see more and be more aware, it slows us down and brings our animal instincts into control.

> As we train ourselves to see more and be more aware, it slows us down and brings our animal instincts into control.

Once again, the appetite for food is a metaphor for other appetites. As we gain the "lightness" of a perceptive, observant attitude, we lose "weight" and become a higher type of being.

REALLY SEEING

I had an aunt who was a nationally acclaimed poet and who sought to teach me the tricks of her trade when I was a child. I remember one autumn day she pointed at a bright tree and said, "What do you see?"

"A tree," I answered.

"Yes, but what do you *see*?" she said.

"Well, I see red and orange leaves."

"Good," she said, "and what else?"

She taught me that day to see the patterns in the bark, the delicate flow in the movement of the branches, the imagined intertwining roots underground that give nourishment and balance. When our conversation was over, I saw the tree in a whole new light—and both the "whole" and the "light" began to have double meanings. She helped me write a poem about the tree, to capture and remember the new perspectives and the new awareness.

That tree was in our front yard, and I never looked at it the same again. I remember walking past it one day on my way home from sixth grade and thinking, "That tree is a miracle! It is worth more than our house!" I had learned that the best things in life really are free—free to those who learn to really see them and truly appreciate them.

BLESSINGS

Amazing benefits come from a more poetic soul. Here are a few things that we become:

- More aware; less gluttonous
- More appreciative; less greedy
- More interested in aesthetics; less interested in self-gratification

It is telling that in our fast, competitive, greedy world, the first question we often ask those we meet is "What do you do?"

I would rather ask someone "What do you see?" or "What do you feel?" or even "What do you love?"

Feelings and observations (and joy, too, for that matter) come in moments. Becoming more aware and more appreciative of those moments of joy is the key to happiness. Awareness of joyful moments gives us the perspective and peace that allow us to slow down a little and gain better control of the appetites to hurry, to obtain, to win, to control, and to gain power.

> The first question we often ask those we meet is "What do you do?"
>
> I would rather ask someone "What do you see?" or "What do you feel?" or even "What do you love?"

The best way I know to increase awareness and appreciation of moments is to try to capture them in small, private poems. It might be just a line or two, and it can be completely private. Challenge yourself to create at least one short verse about at least one moment of awareness and joy each day. It will do three amazing things for you: (1) help you remember pleasant moments (and thus retain their joy for longer), (2) cause you to look harder for those moments and thus recognize more of them, and (3) make you more attuned to the quality and the blessings that surround you and thus less susceptible to the pull of petty, personal appetites.

At the risk of embarrassment and further revealing of my very amateur status as a poet, let me close this chapter with a few more of my own little daily verses, the purpose not being to lay claim to any poetic talent but rather to show you that it takes no talent to attempt!

Five grandkids,
Ten eyes, four colors,
Billy's chocolate brown, Tawni's tan/green,
Holly's violet blue, and the last four, two on each twin,
The color of morning sky.

Morning sleeper, arms flung up overhead,
Sweet face of virtue,
Soft snores of peace.
Watching your morning slumber
Makes it worth it to get up first.

Funeral,
Grief, heavy and sweet,
Choked with love, bearing down on hope.
Celebrate a life and recommit to more love.

A storm over the lake,
The wet smell of sagebrush,
Stop; use eyes and nose better for just a minute
because it's a moment.

Early morning, pastoral summer grass, backlit lawn
Through my own plantation shutters as I
Relearn the book of James.
Ahhh, solitary morning meditation.

The rhythm-laughter of memories
Rubbing the pleasant traction of
Renewed acquaintance,
Just a simple dinner with old friends; years melt away
And friendship remains.

CHAPTER 19

THE MENTAL BRIDLE

Compare to Chapter 9

Chapter 9, if you recall, talked of bits and bridles and quoted James the apostle: "We put bits in the horses' mouths, that they may obey us; and we turn about their whole body." To become "perfect men," he said, we must be "able also to bridle" our bodies, our expressions, our appetites.

A horse is the perfect metaphor because of its beauty and power and its ability to serve us and make our lives better and more filled with grace. We can be hurt by horses only when we fail to control them—and the way to control them is not to drug them or bind them but to bridle them.

Like we discussed before, our passions and our appetites are not our enemies but our energies. They can be our motivators.

But only with the bridle!

Truly, the last thing we should want to do with our appetite for food, or for sex, or for any of God's gifts is to dull it, to subdue it, to tie it up or hobble it so it loses its beauty and strength and passion, or to kill it. Your brain is the bridle, and your mental commitment to eat half as much twice as slowly is the bit that can gradually come to feel natural and accepted in the mouth!

YOUR BRAIN IS THE BRIDLE

The brain can control the body like a bridle controls a horse. Work the metaphor a little deeper: Just having a bridle (or a brain) is not enough. We must learn how to use it to control the horse (the appetite). We must practice and learn the skills of riding; we must develop the strength of will that puts us in charge. Then and only then does the horse or the appetite serve us and give us joy.

> Without the bridle and the developed skill to use it, we spiral down toward danger and death; with it, we climb upward toward the confidence and happiness of a wonderful ride.

Each chapter in the physical diet was on an idea or technique or practice that can give us a better bridle and more skill in using it to control the food appetite. Each of those methods, from sipping and savoring to fasting and poetic awareness, can help us learn to bridle all of our other physical and mental appetites as well.

What is at stake? Everything! Without the bridle and the developed skill to use it, we spiral down toward danger and death; with it, we climb upward toward the confidence and happiness of a wonderful ride.

With discipline and the will that is gained through practice and effort, we lift ourselves higher toward peace and joy. Without it, we plummet toward obsessions that lead to addictions and other deep unhappiness.

And the difference is the bridle!

A bridle actually has three parts. First, the halter or head harness fits snugly over the horse's head to hold everything in place. Second, the bit goes into the back of the horse's mouth so he can be pulled up short and stopped. Third, the reins allow the rider to turn or direct the horse's action and movement.

Our will and discipline, to be effective, need the same parts. First, we need to understand our appetites so we can fit our discipline to its dimensions. We need to understand the purposes and makeups and best uses of food, wealth, power, sex—of every desire or urge we have—and fit them into what we know of the Lord's will and the purpose of life. Second, we need to be able to absolutely deny or stop our appetites from pulling us in directions we know are contrary to what is right or good for ourselves and those around us. And third, we need to turn or transform the directions our appetites take us from negative to positive. These are what we must turn from:

- Turn our passion for food away from gluttony and toward serious interest in nutrition and gourmet enjoyment
- Turn our sexual desires away from pornography or perversion or selfish gratification and toward commitment and fidelity and ultimate oneness with our now or future spouse
- Turn our materialistic interests from envy or covetousness or greed toward unselfish magnification of stewardships
- Turn our power appetite from Machiavellian control and domination toward win-win interdependence

Like the little Transformer toys that kids play with, which, with a few twists and rotations, go from a man to a spaceship or a race car, we can transform our passions from dangerous (to ourselves and to others) masters into obedient and highly beneficial (and joy-giving) servants.

You already have the bridle. God has given it to each of us just as he has given us the horse. It is up to us to use it. It is up to us to learn to ride!

CHAPTER 20

REVIEW OF THE PRINCIPLES AND PRACTICES OF THE MENTAL DIET

Compare to Chapter 10

Let's take a quick look back at what we have covered so far in the mental part of the Half Diet. It is important to have the principles and practices well in mind in order to implement both the physical and mental parts of the diet and to help prepare us to comprehend the spiritual parts of the diet that are still to come. The following lists come from the concepts and challenges outlined in Chapters 11–19. You may also want to compare these mental principles and practices with the physical principles and practices that were reviewed back in Chapter 10.

Fourteen simple principles of the mental diet:

1. Active, engaged thinking about a broad range of ideas and things is good for the brain, as are mental games and puzzles.

2. Our mental appetites, our curiosities, and even our lusts can work for us, but they often work against us because they do not know when to stop or how to direct themselves.

3. At least half of what we take into our brains is junk—which is detrimental rather than beneficial to our minds. By limiting and being discerning about what we let into our brains—"eating half," as it were—we can cause ourselves to gradually gravitate toward thoughts and ideas that are twice as good. (Our minds, denied the addicting fluff that surrounds us, will begin to appreciate and even demand a higher quality of thought.)

4. By thinking more deliberately and taking our time on important conclusions and decisions, we cast aside stress and pressure and make fewer mistakes.

5. The more sensual attention we pay to our surroundings, the more interesting and pleasing they become.

6. The most important and most enjoyable things we can think about are our relationships.

7. Thirsting for the clear light of truth will lead to the gift of discernment.

8. A mind that is full of light and truth will ask for and be satisfied with fewer small-minded stimulations (everything from small talk to mindless television).

9. Letting the brain have downtime and rest periodically can cleanse, rejuvenate, and recalibrate capacity.

10. Mental and spiritual awareness is heightened and sharpened by meditation.

11. Regulating the output of mental exercise (creating, planning, solving) is as important as regulating the input (reading, watching,

listening). With some effort and attention, everyone can find a form of mental exercise he or she loves. Mental puzzle- or problem-solving, because of the endorphins it produces, can become a positive addiction.

12. Service and giving to others takes our minds off of ourselves and increases our JQ (Joy Quotient) as well as our IQ.

13. Poetry or other artistic outlets enhance awareness, slow us down, orient us to quality, and increase our discipline.

14. The horse-and-bridle metaphor can help us visualize and implement better control of all of our appetites.

Seven simple practices of the mental diet:

1. Focus on your three stewardships: your family, your work, and yourself (e.g., character).

2. Mentally create a "choose-to-do" for each of these three stewardships every day—something you don't have to do but choose to do for the benefit of that stewardship. Plan these before listing the "have-to-dos."

3. Slow down. Walk more slowly, eat more slowly, think more about what you are feeling, and be consciously aware of each of your five senses and what they are telling you.

4. Visualize. Create things mentally before you do them.

5. Stop thinking and doing once in a while. Just relax, do nothing, think nothing. Take naps. Push your reset button.

6. Exercise your mind through creating or solving. Paint, write, do crosswords, or engage in the mental exercise of your choice at least three times a week.

7. Conserve resources, don't waste, and find a service project or charity that you can become passionate about.

It is fortunate that we use the same word for the losing of weight and for the gaining of illumination, because it enables this chapter to end with a single promise that comes to those who implement the physical diet and the mental diet. The promise is: "You will become *lighter!*"

Now, consider the same questions we asked about the physical diet principles and practices: Do you believe these fourteen principles? Can you implement these seven practices? Let your belief in the principles expand your motivation to implement the practices.

Work at it! Don't give up! The mental results will be as obvious as the physical results.

It is fortunate that we use the same word for the losing of weight and for the gaining of illumination, because it enables this chapter to end with a single promise that comes to those who implement the physical diet and the mental diet. The promise is: "You will become *lighter!*"

REDUCING IT ALL DOWN TO FIVE BAD HABITS AND FIVE GOOD HABITS

Like the physical diet, the mental diet can be broken down into a simple list of bad habits to avoid or overcome and a mirror-image list of good habits to develop. Our minds, like our bodies, are durable and resilient and can bounce back from both abuse and lack of use, but there are certain bad mental habits that can wear our brains down and eventually weaken them.

Again, like the bad physical habits, these are negative practices that can creep up on us, that are subtle, and even that seem fairly harmless. They are not habits like using drugs or glue-sniffing or things that everyone knows will fry their brains. They are behaviors that we kind of slide into, that become our "norms," and that work against the full and best functioning of our minds.

There are five of these bad habits:

1. *Screen hypnosis.* Have you noticed the trance that large and small screens put children into? Whether they are watching a cartoon or playing a game on a smartphone, their eyes glaze over and they become oblivious to the environment (and the people) around them. Virtual reality becomes their reality, and actual reality fades from view. But guess what—it's not only kids. The biggest of all the bad mental habits for adults in today's world is falling often and for lengthy periods into screen hypnosis. Needing to be endlessly entertained. Keeping track of seemingly endless social media. Addiction that demands our attention and takes us away from what matters more.

2. *Device handcuffs.* Like food all around us, data is all around us and we consume too much of it. Instead of controlling them, we begin to be used and controlled by our devices. We forget we have the power to turn them off and to call them to us only when we want them to serve us.

3. *Ongoing, unexamined routine.* We spend too much time going through mindless motions. What if what Socrates said millennia ago is true (and it is)—that "the unexamined life is not worth living"? Many of us have a problem. "Examining" involves asking "Why?" Why do we spend our days the way we do? Why do we work the hours we do? Why do we prioritize the wrong things? Why don't our real priorities match up with how we allocate our thought and our effort? Why do we do things the same way? Why do we want more of so many things? Why aren't we more selective and simplified?

4. *Hurrying and rushing.* Thoreau asked, "Why should we be in such desperate haste to succeed, and in such desperate enterprises? If a man does not keep pace with his companions, perhaps it is because he hears a different drummer. Let him step to the music which he hears, however measured or far away."[21] We blame it on

the pace of the world around us. We blame it on keeping up with the neighbors. We blame it on business. But the fact is that we can slow ourselves down. And we should.

5. *Mental inactivity.* We live in a world where it is too easy to sit back mentally and wait for something to challenge or entertain us rather than challenging ourselves to try new things, learn new fields, or test our minds. And a sedentary mind weakens and goes flabby as surely as a sedentary body.

Bad habits come on us gradually. No one sets out to be hassled and rushed. We don't consciously become slaves to our smartphones or TV zombies. And none of us want to be stuck in ruts of routines, to develop brain-destroying mental addictions or brain-atrophying mental laziness. They creep up on us.

But the way to change all this is not slow or gradual. The best correction is an immediate one. Substitute your bad habits with good ones, and the antitheses of these five bad mental habits are the five good mental habits that form the core of the mental Half Diet:

1. *The screen-selectivity-and-device-discipline habit.* Don't turn on a TV until you are ready to watch it, or a computer or smartphone until you are ready to use it. Don't use any large or small screen for companionship. Before you press any power button, ask "Why?" Why are you turning it on right now? Is it the most important and most useful and most relevant thing you can do right now?

2. *The Sunday-session habit.* Nothing disrupts stale routine and eliminates hypnotic screen time-wasting than personal goal-setting and future planning. The best goal- and plan-creation habit I have ever seen involves carving out some quiet time every Sunday for this sequence: (a) think through long-term goals for family, work, and personal needs, keeping track of those goals in a personal journal; (b) review yearly goals that lead toward those long-term goals; (c) refine monthly goals within the same framework or set monthly goals on the first Sunday of the month; and (d) plan the week

ahead within the context of the monthly, yearly, and long-term goals just reviewed. Once personal goals and plans have been set and written down, you will be mentally stimulated and motivated and far less likely to fall into a time-wasting routine and passive couch-potatoing.

3. *The take-charge-of-the-day habit.* The whole idea with these good habits is to become more proactive and less reactive. The mental diet is about conditioning your mind to work for you. Longer-term goal setting helps mightily with this, but where the rubber really hits the road is in how you structure and plan each individual day. And even though large chunks of your day are not fully in your control (work, duties, responsibilities), you can still be in control by doing three things in the morning (or the night before) as you plan your day: (a) Before you list your "have-to-dos," take five minutes to decide on three "choose-to-dos"—one for your family, one for your work, and one for yourself. These are things you don't have to do, needs you can meet, little things that make a difference. (b) Find at least two "serendipities" each day. Serendipity is something you didn't plan but chance upon because you are aware and observant and looking for it. It could be something as simple as taking a moment to watch a sunset or trying a new route on your drive home. Write the serendipities down. (c) Pause briefly three times a day to pray or meditate—once in the morning as you get up, once either at lunch or at the end of the workday, and once before you retire for the evening. Use these three moments to slow down, to breathe, to refocus.

4. *The name-and-poem habit.* During that last "pause moment" just before bed, think back over the day and give the day a name based on the best thing that happened or the most important thing you noticed. Write the day's name on your calendar. And on Sunday, as a new week starts, write in your private journal a brief poem about the week just past, recalling and recording what you felt, what you liked, whom you loved. Not every day or every week

will go as you wish, but there will always be good things within them, and capturing them with a name or a poem will magnify their joy and make you more aware.

5. *The education-and-brain-exercise habit.* At least once a week, do some kind of brain exercise—a crossword, Sudoku, or any of the wide array of puzzles and brain stretchers available on apps or online.

> These habits take commitment and discipline, but they can actually be developed and become part of your life rather quickly! If you do something for twenty-one straight days, it becomes a habit.

These habits take commitment and discipline, but they can actually be developed and become part of your life rather quickly! If you do something for twenty-one straight days, it becomes a habit.

Even as you begin to master the principles, the practices, and the habits of the mental Half Diet, you may start to understand that just as the physical diet prepared you for the mental, so the mental can be a precursor to the ultimate diet of the whole soul, the whole spirit. But be prepared as you move on, because while the mental diet was essentially a parallel to the physical diet, the spiritual diet is, in many ways, the exact opposite of both.

GIVING FREE REIN TO YOUR SPIRIT

I n a three-act play, we need two intermissions. This short break is to briefly review where we have been so far and to set the stage for a spiritual diet that is fundamentally different from its physical and mental counterparts.

The first ten chapters laid out the physical Half Diet. Based on extensive feedback from the thousands who have tried it, I know that different individuals found different ways to get into the diet—different "entry points" that appealed to them and got them going. Some found the "sip and savor" approach appealing; others liked the "give back" or "water first" or "poetry diet" techniques. Then, from whatever starting point appealed to them, they went on to embrace the rest of the diet. And once they were into it, it was the personal results—the actuality of the weight they had lost—that motivated them to keep going.

But the promise of the diet is more than physical, more than the loss of weight. The promise is that you will be "lighter" not only in terms of weight but in terms of illumination and optimism—lighter in mind and in mood as well as in body. We moved on, in the next ten chapters, to the mental diet, applying every "type" learned about how our bodies work to

If our mental faculties can bridle and control the physical appetites, what is it that can bridle and control the mental appetites? The answer, of course, is the spiritual faculties.

our brains—to the way we think and the way we live as well as to the way we eat.

Much of the mental Half Diet has been the realization that awareness and perspective can lift us above our urges and appetites. The more aware we are, the less greedy. The broader our perspective, the less gluttonous we become.

And it was Christ, of course, who taught us to elevate all truth and all commandments from the physical to the mental. In place of "Don't kill," he said, "Don't be angry." And instead of "Don't commit adultery," he said, "Don't lust."

Essentially, then, physical appetites are controlled with mental attitudes and disciplines. If we sip and savor, concentrating (with our minds) on the taste and joy and quality of eating, we bring the physical appetite to eat under our mental control. The horse-and-bridle metaphor works at every level. By bridling the horse's head, we control his body. There are also social/emotional/mental appetites, lusts, and passions that can destroy us if we let them have their way and take control of our lives. They can work for us or against us depending on which way we lead them—on how we use our bridle. As the New Testament says, "Behold, we put bits in the horses' mouths, that they may obey us; and we turn about their whole body."

So here is the next question: if our mental faculties can bridle and control the physical appetites, what is it that can bridle and control the mental appetites? The answer, of course, is the spiritual faculties. Just as we must elevate our physical appetites to the mental level in order to bridle them, we must elevate our mental appetites to the spiritual level in order to control them.

THREE LEVELS OF LIFE

These three levels represent three completely different ways of thinking and of being. When we live on the physical level, we are animals—obeying our instincts, appetites, urges, and lusts and following the law of the jungle. When we live on the mental level, we are rational, decision-making human beings—analyzing, making conscious choices based on what we think is good and what we think makes sense, and following the laws of logic and of men. When we live on the spiritual level, we are children of God—seeking his will, tapping into his power, striving to do what is right, and living by his law. The problem with our perception is that the physical is more obvious than the mental, and the spiritual is often the hardest of the three to see. When you look at another person, what do you see? What do you perceive? What are you interested in? Are you inclined to see a person's body and appearance, or his mind, or his spirit? Oh, that we could see the spirit more easily.

In India, the standard greeting (instead of "Hello" or "How are you?") is "Namaste," which, literally translated, means "I bow to the divine spark within you." Oh, that we really could see that part of each person we meet.

In India, the standard greeting (instead of "Hello" or "How are you?") is "Namaste," which, literally translated, means "I bow to the divine spark within you." Oh, that we really could see that part of each person we meet.

Appetites can be identified and classified (and potentially controlled) on these same three levels. Physical appetites such as food and sex, when they are left to the physical, become gluttony and perversion. When they are bridled by the mental, they provide us with and allow us to express nourishment and love and joy.

Mental/emotional/social appetites (such as those for power, control, popularity, and wealth), if they are given their head, can run away to become selfish obsessions for dominion, materialism, and fame—or they can be bridled and transformed into the spiritual desire for stewardship, wisdom, contribution, and discipleship.

> Spiritual appetites are all good. True spiritual desires are always for aspects and dimensions of God's will. Spiritual appetites are for truth, wisdom, faith, insight, righteousness, and eternal awareness and perspective.

And here is the secret and the differentiation: spiritual appetites are all good. True spiritual desires are always for aspects and dimensions of God's will. Spiritual appetites are for truth, wisdom, faith, insight, righteousness, and eternal awareness and perspective.

Unlike physical appetites (which, unchecked, will always harm us) and mental appetites (which can result in bad or good depending on our skill with the bridle), spiritual appetites (the urges and longings and desires of our spirits) all draw us toward home and toward God. The trick (and the ultimate goal of the Half-Diet Diet) is first to put the physical under the control of the mental bridle and then to transform our mental appetites into spiritual ones, where the bridle becomes the will of God's mind rather than of our own.

During the course of the next ten chapters, we will progress and elevate to the spiritual diet. But as we do, remember that many of the benefits and dividends are still physical and mental. The better you get at the mental diet, the more you will control your physical weight, and the better you get at the spiritual diet, the more you will be able to control your mind. The principles remain the same on all levels. And the techniques and control methods you have learned and continue to practice for the physical and mental diets are good training, as well as good metaphors, for the spiritual diet. But, as we shall see, the spiritual diet supersedes and transforms all other diets.

ACT III

THE SPIRITUAL
HALF DIET

When I am asked to speak on the Half Diet or on controlling appetites, I often use my hand's five fingers to symbolize the five facets or the five dimensions of our physical, mental, emotional, social, and spiritual selves. This allows me to point out that, ideally, the spiritual dimension is the thumb—the one that can work with each of the others, the one that can make the others functional and effective, the one that we want in charge and in control of the other four. Turning my hand upside down, I try to illustrate this idea by holding the thumb above and in charge of the other four.

Your own hand can become a reminder that your physical, mental, social, and emotional selves can be thought of as the servant fingers, directed and controlled by the spiritual thumb, which is different in kind from the fingers because its movement can be directed and inspired by a higher force.

Developing and honing that spiritual direction gives you the ultimate control of your negative and potentially harmful physical, social, emotional, and mental appetites. Keep the thumb-and-fingers metaphor in mind as we shift paradigms in the next ten chapters.

The spiritual diet is more than a better bridle—it is a shift of horses. And the spiritual horse, as you will see, does not need a bridle at all. It is a horse you can trust, a horse that knows the way home. It is a horse that was sent to you and that can, if well ridden, transform its rider to resemble its sender.

There is always some risk in writing in a spiritual paradigm. The risk is someone saying, "Why do you assume that everyone is a believer? Is religious or spiritual faith a prerequisite for reading this book?"

It is a risk I'm willing to take, because the Half Diet does not reach its full meaning or effect without the spiritual dimension—and I am also somewhat emboldened by the 2011 public opinion poll numbers that reveal that more than 90 percent of Americans profess a belief in God.[22]

But back to the question: is faith a prerequisite for reading this book? Absolutely not. If you read Act I as a physical diet and found it reasonable and effective, that is enough—more than enough. And if you found some added benefit in the mental Half Diet of Act II, so much the better.

And if the first two acts made you curious about the third, read on.

CHAPTER 21

FOCUSING ON GOD'S WILL—CHOOSING HIS HALF

Compare to Chapters 1 and 11

The introduction you just read compared the spiritual diet to a new and completely different horse. Most horses need a bridle to keep them in check, but the spiritual horse needs no bridle at all. Although the terminology of it may sound a little unfamiliar, the basic spiritual appetite is to discover and to do God's will. There is a spirit in each of us that is drawn toward home and toward light. Yet that spirit is encased in a mortal body that, according to God's plan, is filled with physical and mental or emotional appetites that, if unbridled, pull us in other directions. Thus our mortality is subject to the tugs and forces of the opposing, dark side.

Bridling these mortal appetites and pulling them into control can fill us with strengthening love that enables us to catch up to and ultimately swing across and mount the spiritual horse. Doing this is both the test and the glorifying challenge of life on this earth.

Mortality is essentially a binary situation that offers, ultimately, only two basic choices: light or darkness. Each choice moves us either toward God or away from him.

Everything that entices us to good is from him. Everything that leads us away is not. The spiritual Half Diet takes on new meaning as we focus on choosing *the right half*—the true half—the light half.

> In the physical and mental diets, the challenge was to control our urges and our appetites. In the spiritual diet, the challenge is to give control to God.

This is a huge paradigm shift. In the physical and mental diets, the challenge was to control our urges and our appetites. In the spiritual diet, the challenge is to give control to God. In the ultimate spiritual reality, since God owns all, the only thing we have to give to him is our agency. When we truly and fully do that, when we have relinquished all control, we no longer need the bridle, because we have climbed on a very different kind of horse which, unbridled, takes us away in God's direction.

The physical and mental horses still live in our pasture, and we must ride them, too, because they are in our charge and we love them and we appreciate what they can do for us. As we ride them, always with a bridle and always in control, we are filled with more and more love, and over time they become better and more manageable horses because they are ridden well and because they share the same pasture with the spiritual horse, which can influence them.

WHO IS THE MASTER?

It is hard to know the right name for this total paradigm shift to the third horse. Submission? Consecration? Elevation? Whatever it is, it changes everything. We move directly away from self-determination and control—the very things the whole world seems to be seeking. To illustrate the drama of this shift, compare some lines from the oft-quoted poem "Invictus" with the corresponding lines from a spiritual rebuttal mirror poem, "The Soul's Captain (The Answer)," written by a man named Orson Whitney.

Invictus
by William E. Henley

Out of the night that covers me,
Black as the Pit from pole to pole,
I thank whatever gods may be
For my unconquerable soul.
In the fell clutch of circumstance,
I have not winced nor cried aloud.
Under the bludgeonings of chance
My head is bloody, but unbowed.

Beyond this place of wrath and tears
Looms but the Horror of the shade,
And yet the menace of the years
Finds, and shall find, me unafraid.

It matters not how strait the gate,
How charged with punishments the scroll,
I am the master of my fate:
I am the captain of my soul.

The Soul's Captain (The Answer)
by Orson F. Whitney

Art thou in truth? Then what of him
Who bought thee with his blood?
Who plunged into devouring seas
And snatched thee from the flood?

Who bore for all our fallen race
What none but him could bear—
The God who died that man might live,
And endless glory share?

Of what avail thy vaunted strength,
Apart from his vast might?
Pray that his Light may pierce the gloom,
That thou mayest see aright.

Men are as bubbles on the wave,
As leaves upon the tree.
Thou, captain of thy soul, forsooth
Who gave that place to thee?

Free will is thine—free agency
To wield for right or wrong;
But thou must answer unto him
To whom all souls belong.

Bend to the dust that head "unbowed,"
Small part of Life's great whole!
And see in him, and him alone,
The Captain of thy soul.

There is great folly in believing we are the captains or the masters of our destiny. So much of life and its circumstances is so far beyond our control. We are dependent on God and interdependent on each other in so many ways. And in the Christian perspective, we have been bought and purchased—ransomed—by the one who has all control, and in this we should find our greatest rejoicing.

And what errors we would make if we were really in charge—mistakes that might rob us of the very things we were sent here to gain.

The eat-half diet, in its spiritual phase, becomes the *choose-half* diet. We choose God's half; we choose the light. What we give away is the dark half, the natural man, the world. And we give to God the only thing we really have, the only thing we can ever claim to own—our agency!

In the next chapter, we will explore further how obsession with control can suck the quality and the joy out of our lives and make us forget the true captain of our souls. And we will think more about the magnificent and adventuresome ride we are in for as we give the spiritual horse his head and commit ourselves to going wherever God takes us.

> The eat-half diet, in its spiritual phase, becomes the *choose-half* diet.
>
> We choose God's half; we choose the light. What we give away is the dark half, the natural man, the world.

CHAPTER 22

WHAT SLOWING DOWN AND TUNING YOUR SPIRIT WILL DO FOR YOU

Compare to Chapters 2 and 12

One of the hundreds of endorsement letters I received abut the first edition of this book, when I was still authoring it as "Dr. Bridell," made an interesting connection between the physical, mental, and spiritual aspects of the Half Diet:

Dear Dr. Bridell,

I wanted you to know how well your diet works and the freedom it provides. I was on my way to the doctor to look into gastric bypass. I was that desperately crazy to lose weight. Then I talked at length with a long-distance friend, and she said to look into your "mysterious" diet. It works, she said. And so it does.

In five months, I am down over ninety pounds—forty to go. I have not suffered or felt deprived as I have changed everything about how I eat. Half of everything, lots of water, swimming because I love to and I do not care how I look in a bathing suit, walks when I want to, which have turned into daily. (My chocolate lab who walks with me has lost ten pounds, which she needed to do.)

My husband has Parkinson's disease, and he is now much healthier because he is along for the ride, as he says. And the interesting thing is that as we have become more disciplined, or more "bridled," we have also become more spiritual. We find it easier and more natural to read the Bible and to pray, and our whole outlook has become more contemplative and spirit oriented.

The Half Diet works. It is wonderful. Thank you so much for restoring my spirit through your "mysterious" self.

A friend, admirer, and more,

Shalom

JC

The letter provides an interesting segue between the physical/mental diets and the spiritual one. It sounds as though this reader, in addition to her dramatic physical results, has been invited by the diet to a more spiritual place where scripture and prayer and all things of the spirit have become more natural, more prominent, and more prioritized.

PHYSICAL CONTROLLED BY MENTAL CONTROLLED BY SPIRITUAL

The promise of the physical diet (remember from Chapter 2) was that as you cut the quantity intake of food by half, your body will start desiring and demanding better quality from what you do put in your mouth. Junk and fast food will look less appetizing; vegetables and fruit will look better and better. Remember, from Chapter 12, that the same principle works with your mind. As you cut some of the trash and non-nourishing stuff out of your life, your mind will gradually begin to appreciate and even crave more quality in your activities, your entertainment, your interests, and your relationships.

In the physical diet, the key to eating half as much is to eat twice as slowly. Slowing down the way you eat (smaller bites, more chewing, savoring each morsel) lets your body reward you by enjoying food more, craving quality, and getting fitter and stronger. In our intellectual life, we need to do the same thing. As you slow down and simplify the way you live and the way you think, your brain rewards you by producing better ideas and purer thoughts, noticing more beauty, and becoming more perceptive and more aware.

Remember the advice from Chapter 12: "If you can slow down eating, you start to feel that you can slow down other things. Let that kiss for your loved one linger a little longer. Look into a person's eyes and hold their hand a half second longer when you greet them. Sit down and take a look around you for a moment before you start a job at work."

> Slowing down our brains clarifies and sharpens our thoughts and opens up the space and the channels into which and through which inspiration and spiritual nourishment flows.

Do you begin to see the progression? Slowing down physically produces mental benefits, and slowing down mentally produces spiritual blessings. Slowing down our bodies helps us control our physical appetites; we lose weight and become more cerebral, our minds more alert and more alive. Slowing down our brains clarifies and sharpens our thoughts and opens up the space and the channels into which and through which inspiration and spiritual nourishment flows.

Scripture advises us to "be still and know."[23] The simple fact is that inspiration and enlightenment cannot come to a hurried, frazzled, multi-focused mind. Quieting the mind, slowing it down, and making it still and receptive is the key to inviting and feeling the Spirit.

The hectic world we live in today is the hardest environment there has ever been for that kind of slowing and stillness. All of our senses are almost constantly bombarded by noise, by lights, by commercial messages, by endless information that exceeds by a million times what we could ever take in. Nature and the quiet countryside which inspired and nourished our grandparents is virtually gone, replaced with a "virtual reality" that is so superficial that it reflects away the Spirit rather than inviting and absorbing it.

Yet the Spirit, when it is within us, somehow holds the swirling stress at bay and creates in us an island of calm awareness. Parley P. Pratt, in his book *Key to the Science of Theology*, described the effects of the Holy Spirit as a gift that "adapts itself to all these organs and attributes. It quickens all the intellectual faculties, increases, enlarges, expands and purifies all the natural passions and affections; and adapts them, by the gift of wisdom, to their lawful use. It inspires, develops, cultivates and matures all the fine toned sympathies, joys, tastes, kindred feelings and affections of our nature. It inspires virtue, kindness, goodness, tenderness, gentleness and charity. It developes beauty of person, form and features. It tends to health, vigour, animation and social feeling. It developes and invigorates all the faculties of the physical and intellectual man. It strengthens, invigorates, and gives tone to the nerves. In short, it is, as it were, marrow to the bone, joy to the heart, light to the eyes, music to the ears, and life to the whole being."[24]

Quite a gift! But the chicken-and-egg question is: does the Spirit calm us and clear us and slow us, or does our own slow, still calmness attract the Spirit to us? The answer is both! It works both ways. Our physical, mental, and spiritual parts have profound effects on each other.

If we rush and hurry physically, we stress and frazzle our thought process, making it erratic and scattered. And vice versa.

A frantic physical and mental pace creates within us a scattered, unreceptive spirit. And vice versa.

But when we consciously slow ourselves down, body and mind, moving more slowly, thinking more deliberately, finding some time and place for solitude, the Spirit finds us more easily and dwells with us. And vice versa—when we pray for and feel the Spirit, it slows us down, makes us more aware, and transforms physical/mental appetites into spiritual ones that lift us toward God rather than pulling us down and away.

So besides eating more slowly, moving more slowly, and thinking more deliberately, make a conscious effort to pray more slowly (listening more, thinking more), to breathe and meditate more deeply, to read one verse of scripture but think about it as long as it would normally take you to read ten.

When you bridle and control and slow down your body, it rewards you by shedding unwanted weight and by beginning to crave good things rather than junk. When you bridle the mind, it rewards you by becoming more discerning and more creative and by gravitating to the light. And when you care for and focus on the needs of your spirit, taking time to listen while you pray and "wait upon the Lord,"[25] your spirit rewards you by connecting with God and causing you to desire what he desires for you.

THE IMPORTANCE OF THE SABBATH DAY IN THE HALF-DIET DIET

The Sabbath is the Lord's renewal and calibration tool. It can reset our bodies as well as our souls. It can provide the reassessment that keeps us on course to progress that is regular, measurable, and consistent. It adds new meaning to the truth that "The Sabbath was made for man, not man for the Sabbath."[26]

God gave us this day, and the whole concept of a sabbatical, to bless us. He made us in such a way that we function best when we shut down and reset every seven days. He exemplified this pattern when he made the earth in a sequence of six creative periods and then rested on the seventh. And he made the earth itself to function in this same pattern, so that when land is given a "sabbatical" and allowed to lie fallow and rest each seventh year, it becomes more productive and more vital. Many of the gifts promised for Sabbath-day observance relate to the earth, and "the fullness" of it will be ours if we observe the Sabbath.[27]

The Sabbath is the Lord's renewal and calibration tool. It can reset our bodies as well as our souls. It can provide the reassessment that keeps us on course to progress that is regular, measurable, and consistent.

The key ingredient of a well-observed Sabbath is worship, which we usually think of as a spiritual and mental process. But our observation can also be partially physical. We can worship with our bodies by fasting and by purging and purifying them. Putting the body to rest can activate and energize and give focus to the spirit.

A good summary of what we should try to do on the Sabbath can be made up of "re-" words: rest, rejuvenate, renew, reset, re-create, review, recalibrate, and replenish.

Some of us use Sunday brunches and dinners as a time to feast, even to gorge. And some of this, particularly when surrounded by family, is positive. But on a more regular basis, we ought to do just the opposite. Simplify your food on Sundays. Eat very slowly, and eat only the best and healthiest food. Prepare food simply and with singleness of heart. If possible, prepare it on the day before the Sabbath. Eat little or nothing before attending church or synagogue. If you are Christian, let the emblems of the sacrament of the Lord's Supper be the first food you partake of on a Sunday.

SUNDAY PRACTICES

The essential pattern is to work for six days and then to use the seventh to rest and to plan for the coming week. Some specific weekly reassessments can also become a powerful part of your physical worship on Sundays:

1. Keep a Sunday journal in which you write the feelings and impressions you have during your worship and prayer.

2. Don't expect dramatic change week by week, but keep track of the steady progress of your eat-half diet. As part of your entry each week, record three things relating to your diet:

- Your weight
- How you have felt physically during the past week
- What foods and types of foods appeal to you most

3. Visualize. Sit back for a few moments, close your eyes, and try to see in your mind both an external and an internal view of your improving physical self:

- Don't be extreme or wildly unrealistic. Don't try to see yourself fifty pounds lighter or perfect in every way, but visualize improvement. See yourself trimmer, healthier, getting stronger. Visualize yourself moving better, eating more slowly, becoming firmer and straighter and more energized.

> Let Sunday be your day of reassessment—spiritually, mentally, and physically. Try to progress from Sunday to Sunday. Have modest but motivating weekly goals.

- Think about the systems within your body and try to see them in your mind's eye. Your digestive system, clear and functional, not weighted down or bloated or at overcapacity, but smooth and efficient. Visualize your circulatory system open and flowing, your breathing and lungs unobstructed, open and easy, your blood oxygenating. Scriptural phrases can create good visualizing images. "Health to thy navel"[28] can prompt positive images of open, flowing, and functioning blood vessels and organs. "Marrow to thy bones"[29] can help you visualize strong immune systems and bones, and so on.

Let Sunday be your day of reassessment—spiritually, mentally, and physically. Try to progress from Sunday to Sunday. Have modest but motivating weekly goals. Ask for help. Become who you believe God wants you to be in tiny steps, one week at a time.

CHAPTER 23

SPIRITUAL SIPPING AND SAVORING

Compare to Chapters 3 and 13

Thinking back to the corresponding physical and mental Half Diets, you will remember these principles: When our food appetite controls us, we rush through meals, gorging ourselves, animal-like, and missing much of the taste and enjoyment. When our other appetites, lusts, and instincts control us (particularly the pervasive appetite for hurry and haste), we rush through our days, missing much of the beauty and subtlety that make life worth living.

When we control our food appetite—sipping, savoring, and smelling our food rather than guzzling, gulping, and gorging it—we can appreciate and taste every morsel. When we control our other appetites (for work, for control, for instant gratification, and especially for haste), we begin to find the moments of joy that are the very purpose of life.

In Chapter 13, you read, "Some people can induce an inner calm simply by commanding themselves to slow down (eating more slowly, walking more slowly, etc.). Others, like a horse straining at the bit, become jumpier and more anxious when forced to go slower. The key for this second type of person is to focus on awareness instead of on slowing down. Do what you need to do: run your errands, check off your list, make your calls, feed the family, get the kids ready, do your work—but while you are doing it, tune in to the present that is all around you. Be aware of smells and sounds. Notice and appreciate things as well as just seeing them. Feel textures, smell aromas, and really taste what you eat. In other words, sip, savor, and smell your life rather than guzzling, gulping, and gorging it."

As with every other aspect of this diet, and every aspect of our appetites, the physical (and the food) serves as a type that helps us better understand, control, and bridle all other instincts, urges, and desires. Once again, as we bridle the physical and the mental, we get to the point where we can develop the beneficial spiritual appetite that needs no bridling and that draws us closer to God.

So how does one apply the principle of sip, savor, and smell to spiritual things? Some applications are obvious: Sip the scriptures; read one verse or one phrase and dwell on it; let it come alive, giving the Spirit time to open your spirit to it. Savor your prayers, taking time to listen and find the power of two-way communication with God. "Smell" and feel the presence of the Spirit and be aware of its calming influence.

RECEIVING

Becoming a good receiver of the gifts of God is a rare skill. We are so busy doing and being and giving (all good things) that we don't have much time or thought left over to simply receive.

Other applications may be less obvious: one who sips and savors is one who appreciates and loves what he receives. Becoming a good receiver of the gifts of God is a rare skill. We are so busy doing and being and giving (all good things) that we don't have much time or thought left over to simply receive.

Becoming a good receiver is a worthy goal, and an increasingly uncommon one. The obvious football analogy comes to mind. No matter how good the quarterback is, passes are seldom complete without a good receiver. Sometimes we get so caught up with the future that we fail to appreciate the present. We get so anxious and consumed with the next thing we want that we fail to appreciate, or even notice, what we already have.

We live at the best time, in the best place, and under the best circumstances of anyone who has ever lived. Most of us have a level of political and personal freedom unknown even to kings in earlier ages. We have mobility and access to the earth and its beauties that no other generation has known. We have more information at our fingertips than whole libraries offered just a decade ago. And yet we do not fully receive these gifts and are not fully grateful for them. "Taking something for granted" is the opposite of being a great and grateful receiver. If we try, we can develop a wonderful spiritual appetite for thankfulness and for awareness of all that we receive.

> When we slow down and find the Spirit's rhythm in our prayers, our scripture study, our meditation, our worship, and our gratitude, we receive the gift of discernment.

When we slow down and sip and savor our food, we receive the gift of taste and enjoyment. When we slow down other appetites and urges and become more observant mentally and more sensitive to the beauty and the people around us, we receive the gift of added awareness and perspective that enhances our joy.

And when we slow down and find the Spirit's rhythm in our prayers, our scripture study, our meditation, our worship, and our gratitude, we receive the gift of discernment, which is one of the great and powerful gifts of God. It can protect us, it can reveal to us the nature and receptivity of the spirits of others, and it can help us make good choices and decisions.

Joy comes in moments, and those moments of joy can come with more frequency and more intensity when we learn to slow down and appreciate and savor God's gifts all around us.

CHAPTER 24

LIVING WATER

Compare to Chapters 4 and 14

One of the truly wonderful stories of the Bible is of Jesus and the woman at the well. He makes her the beautiful promise that he will give to her "living water"[30] and that she will then "never thirst."[31]

What is living water, and how do we obtain it? To try to get at the answer to that spiritual question, let's review the role of water in the physical and mental diets (remembering Chapters 4 and 14): "One of the simplest ways to eat less food is to make less room for it by filling your stomach up with the beautiful, clearing, cleansing, lubricating, hydrating, zero-calorie substance we call water." And: "The same principle and habit works in the mental diet, but the clear water is replaced by clear thought, and the habit we need to develop is to always drink in some of that pure thought before we jump into eating away at any kind of action." Dehydration of body or mind is the enemy to overcome.

So now that we are into the spiritual diet, consider this: how many of us are experiencing "chronic spiritual dehydration"? Like water, we need spiritual nourishment constantly, consistently. We need more of it than we will get if we wait to drink until we are extremely or noticeably thirsty.

Perhaps praying fervently only in crisis or times of deep need is like drinking only when desperately thirsty. Perhaps reading a verse of scripture routinely or robotically once a day is more like taking medicine, one pill a day, than really drinking in the word of God.

The scriptures not only talk about the need for spiritual nourishment; they advocate thirsting for righteousness and thirsting to become more like God.

SPIRITUAL THIRST

Thirst is an appetite, and spiritual thirsting is a spiritual appetite that, like all spiritual appetites, benefits us and needs no bridling. How do we develop and encourage this spiritual thirst, and what is the living water toward which it should be directed?

> Thirst is an appetite, and spiritual thirsting is a spiritual appetite that, like all spiritual appetites, benefits us and needs no bridling.

Spiritual water is spiritual truth; for Christians it is the Gospel and the atonement, and we drink it in by accepting it and by desiring it. Spiritual water is feeling the presence of the Lord. Spiritual hydration comes from having the Holy Spirit in us, coursing through us, refreshing and renewing us.

Just as drinking a full glass of water before eating controls and limits what we eat, drinking in the Spirit before the consumption of the day can control and refine and selectively limit what we take into our minds and our souls as the day progresses. By taking in the good first, we do not later want the bad.

The spiritual application is clear, isn't it?

Clear, but not easy!

It amounts to developing our spiritual appetite and prioritizing it above and before our physical and mental appetites. Here is the application: Before you eat physical food or consume mental food, take a long drink of spiritual, living water. Have your personal prayer and read the scriptures *before* you eat anything in the morning and before you read the newspaper or watch the news or check your social media. In the evenings, drink the spiritual prayer and scripture before you turn on the TV or read a magazine or go online or take in any mental food. Doing so will cause you to want less of the world and to select the best things from it.

If you are a young parent or have circumstances that prevent you from having your spiritual drink in the early mornings and early evenings, find another formula that works better with your schedule, but designate a time and stick to it because spiritual dehydration can set in quickly.

CARRY IT WITH YOU

There is another application or "type" that we can take from the physical diet. Earlier, we said that more water really is the perfect complement to less food all day long. If you get a good water bottle that you like the look and feel of and carry it around with you, sipping becomes a good habit.

Do something similar spiritually. Get a small book of scripture that you like the look and feel of and carry it around with you. Have it with you in the car or set it on your desk, keeping it near you. Let opening it become a habit. I like to do it by seasons. In the winter, I carry an Old Testament; in the spring, I carry the New Testament; in the summer, I carry a favorite spiritually tuned author, like C. S. Lewis; in the fall, I carry a Book of Mormon or a book of scripture from a faith I am less familiar with, like the Buddhist sutras or the Muslim Koran. (I like the small volumes that fit in a purse or briefcase because I like the feel of books—but, of course, an alternative would be an app or site easily accessible on your smartphone.)

Water (physical water, mental water, and spiritual, living water) is a huge key to the spiritual Half Diet. Love it! Drink it! Get results!

CHAPTER 25

EXERCISING FAITH

Compare to Chapters 5 and 15

In the physical diet, it was obvious that exercise had to be an integral part of losing weight and staying fit. Clearly, we have to pay attention to the output of exercise as well as to the intake of food. The mental diet also carries the obvious need of exercise for the brain.

Applying this principle to the spiritual diet is made easy by the wording in many of our sacred books. Think about the terminology of scripture and its use of the metaphors of exercise and exertion and training and discipline:

- "Wrestle against spiritual wickedness"[32]
- "Exercising your faith"[33]
- "And [they] did wax stronger and stronger . . . and firmer and firmer"[34]
- "Pray . . . with all the energy of heart"[35]
- "Evening, and morning, and at noon, will I pray"[36]

It is abundantly and scripturally clear that exertion, regularity, and discipline are required as much in spiritual progression as in physical or mental training.

THE NATURE OF TRAINING

I am reminded of a friend who returned from a humanitarian and missionary expedition to Africa. He commented on how much harder he was finding it to feel spiritually in tune since he had been back at home. It was then pointed out to him that, on his mission, he read the scriptures intently for at least half an hour every morning and prayed hard at least three times a day. Just as a casual toss of a ball a couple of times or a leisurely trot around a track once in a while will never get your body in shape (or cause any weight loss), so a brief little perfunctory prayer now and then or one quick verse of scripture will not bring us into sound and tuned spiritual shape (or cause any positive change from the mindsets and attitudes of the world).

> Exertion, regularity, and discipline are required as much in spiritual progression as in physical or mental training.

Serious training is all about intensity of effort and regularity and discipline of exercise. But more than that, as was emphasized with the physical and mental Half Diets, it is about finding a form of exercise that you love, so that you do it because you want to, not just because you should.

So here are two challenges:

1. Pray and read scripture with regularity and intensity. Pray first thing in the morning and last thing at night, and try for a "middle prayer" as you come home or transition from work or as you find a brief afternoon moment of meditation. Focus the energy of your heart and the intensity of your mind as you pray. Kneel or bow. Apply your energy to your prayer. Take notes on any answers or impressions that come. Visualize a connection to a higher awareness and will your spirit to make a real connection with God as you pray. Also, concentrate hard on some form of scripture or spiritual writing for a few minutes at least once a day. Read what you choose to read with avid interest. After all, what is more important?

2. Find a new and more exciting way to pray and study scripture—
   something that you actually love to do. Try different things. Read by
   subject or by research topic rather than chronologically. Read early
   in the morning or after lunch or some different time than usual.
   Read from a different book of scripture each month or each season.
   Read with a friend on the phone. Find a new and beautiful place to
   read. Try praying right after physical exercise when your mind is
   alert. Pray in your closet (literally, if your closet is big enough . . . or
   find another quiet, private place). If you are married, pray before
   bed with your spouse and make your prayer a meeting with God.
   Have one of you open the verbal prayer and squeeze the other's
   hand when finishing a point of gratitude or request, then have the
   other one pick up the prayer and go back and forth until there are
   no further hand squeezes and the one who did not open closes the
   prayer. Pray with your children and let them talk spontaneously to
   God like they would talk to a wise and loving father. Pray "in your
   fields."[37] Pray while you drive. Pray out loud. Pray sometimes in
   thoughts rather than words. Listen to audio scripture. Find meditation or scriptural apps. Set goals and timetables with other family
   members. Spend the majority of a prayer listening rather than speaking. Take
   notes on what you feel while praying or studying. Keep trying new ways of
   praying and spiritual study and find the ones you love most, the ones that work
   best for you.

> Spend the majority of a prayer listening rather than speaking. Take notes on what you feel while praying or studying.

I have a friend who says, "There is nothing better than a physical
workout. The endorphins get flowing, the blood is pumping, and you feel
so great." I agree and disagree. I agree it feels great, but I disagree that

nothing feels better. The fact is that there is nothing better than a spiritual workout. The spirit gets flowing, and you feel God's love and the emerging clarity of his inspiration.

CHAPTER 26

FASTING, SLOWING, AND FEASTING

Compare to Chapters 6 and 16

n Chapter 16, in the mental diet, we compared physical fasting with mental fasting and concluded that both were essentially about halting our intake of external nourishment (physical food or random mental stimulation) for a period of time so we could turn more within ourselves and be more in touch with our inner selves. We also considered that both physical and mental fasting reduces nervous energy and slows us down.

So what is the spiritual equivalent? What we have already learned is that the spiritual dimension of each aspect of the diet is often the opposite of the physical and the mental. Spiritual appetites do not need a bridle, because they are a horse that we can trust and that will lead us home. While we must bridle and control and often deny our physical and mental appetites, all spiritual appetites draw us toward heaven and God.

So it shouldn't be surprising that the spiritual equivalent of fasting is feasting. It is feasting on the Word. It is feasting on the goodness and generosity and gifts of God and on the richness and wonder of the Spirit.

It shouldn't be surprising that the spiritual equivalent of fasting is feasting. It is feasting on the Word. It is feasting on the goodness and generosity and gifts of God

In the physical and mental diets, we cease our intake (of food or of thought) so that we can clear our bodies and our heads. The fasting and the meditation slow us down and tune us in. But tune us in for what? For the spiritual feast! In the spiritual diet, we need to do just the opposite: stop our output and increase our intake. Stop *doing* for a bit and focus on *receiving.*

In prayer, we can have a spiritual fast/feast by curtailing our output of asking/requesting/pleading for a while and focusing on the intake of listening/receiving/thanksgiving. Feast on the blessings you already have. Consume them by appreciating them. Praise God for his goodness in giving them to you. Feast on your spiritual bounty.

At least once a week, have a special, private, personal prayer that lasts at least ten full minutes during which you ask for nothing; rather, just thank God for all you have, feasting on his blessings. And during your normal prayers, focus more on listening (receiving prompts and impressions and answers, being silent, waiting for insights on the things you have asked). Be silent and in the receiving mode for at least the same amount of time as you are speaking and asking.

The real benefits come when the physical, mental, and spiritual diets are practiced together. This is certainly true with this fasting/slowing principle. As we fast physically, the body benefits through weight loss and system cleansing, the mind becomes clearer, and the spirit becomes more receptive. As we fast mentally (meditation), the body relaxes, the mind resets, and the spirit opens up to the Holy Spirit. And as we feast spiritually, the body is renewed, the mind quickened, and the spirit reborn. We receive these blessings as we apply the principles of fasting and slowing to our bodies, our minds, and our spirits—in other words, to our souls.

CHAPTER 27

THE SPIRITUAL APPETITE FOR GIVING AND SERVING

Compare to Chapters 7 and 17

In earlier chapters, we established the interesting and symbiotic relationship between controlling our consumption and giving to others. In the physical diet, when we got to this giving part, the paradigm shifted and suddenly we were not only talking about caring for our own bodies but also about caring for the bodies of others. In the mental diet, we began to see that a key reason for controlling all of our appetites is that it increases both our capacity and our motivation to care more and to love more.

So, once again, the lesson we must learn with regard to physical and mental appetites is that they must be controlled; when they are, we give ourselves a gift and, at the same time, put ourselves in a position to give gifts to others. The question is: does it work the same way with spiritual appetites?

The key in answering is to remember that physical and mental appetites are the appetites of mortality—of our physical bodies and brains. They will destroy us if they are not controlled but exalt us if they are. These "horses" must be bridled.

Spiritual appetites, on the other hand, are the appetites of eternity, and they save rather than destroy. They are a new kind of horse that needs no bridle and that will take us home. Spiritual appetites come from God and are of God and can make us more like God. They are appetites or desires for all of the things he has: for wisdom and for knowledge, for faith and for peace, for love and for service and for joy. Spiritual passions must be developed and magnified, not controlled or bridled.

> Spiritual appetites are as different from physical or mental appetites as the loaves and fishes of the Lord were from ordinary food.

Spiritual appetites are as different from physical or mental appetites as the loaves and fishes of the Lord were from ordinary food. While ordinary food diminishes and disappears as it is consumed, spiritual food multiplies and increases as it is consumed and as it is given away!

GIVING HIS GIFTS

On the spiritual level, giving becomes giving back. We know that we have been given everything by God, so when we pay a tithing or offering, we are simply returning a percentage to him. When we help or serve in any way, we are simply giving back a tiny morsel of what he has given us.

Giving thus becomes easier, and the more we give, the more we seem to have. In the physical and mental paradigms, we often experience the "scarcity mentality" in which giving to someone else subtracts from what we have. However, in the spiritual paradigm, we can experience the "abundant mentality" in which giving always adds to what we have. As God's servants, it is natural to want to give his gifts. We represent him when we help and serve and give to others.

With a mental or physical appetite, we often find that the more we eat, the more we want, and we move toward addiction. With the spiritual appetite to give and to serve, we learn a new type of positive compulsion or habit. The more we serve, the more we wish to serve and the more blessings we receive. Spiritual appetites turn us outward rather than inward, and, somehow, the more we give, the more we get and the leaner and stronger and more "tuned" we become. The unselfishness of spiritual appetites, particularly the appetite to give and to serve, often overrides the very kind of selfish physical and mental appetites that make us greedy, self-centered, and fat.

In *The Lion, the Witch and the Wardrobe*, the children in the story become so devoted and tuned in to Aslan (the lion that represents Christ) that author C. S. Lewis says they want to be eaten by him, to be swallowed up in his will.[38] Our spiritual appetites are not to eat but to be eaten—to become a part of Christ and his work, to do his will, to become more like him, and to serve him by serving as he served.

Service brings his peace. Giving takes our minds off ourselves and our wants and selfish appetites. When we develop and expand our unselfish spiritual appetites, we have an easier time controlling the selfish appetites of our bodies and minds.

When God says in the New Testament that the purpose of life is to "work out [our] own salvation,"[39] we must realize that the way we work it out is by helping other people with theirs. And real diets—for any of our appetites—are based on the principle that controlling helps us to give and giving helps us to control.

CHAPTER 28

SPIRITUAL POETRY

Compare to Chapters 8 and 18

In the physical and mental Half Diets, we made connections between awareness and discipline. We explored how attempts to see and observe like a poet can help us be more aware of (and thus more demanding about) the quality of what we are taking into our bodies and our minds.

The important thing to realize is that the connection between awareness and appetite control works both ways. When we eat slowly and bridle the appetite for food, we become more aware of the taste, texture, and enjoyment of our small, slow bites. Increasing our awareness and poetic sensitivity slows us down and gives us more control of our urges. It is the same with all appetites. As we bridle them and slow them down, we begin to notice more and appreciate more.

SEEING DEEPER

As mentioned before, instead of "Hello" or "How are you?" the common greeting in India is "Namaste," meaning, "I bow to the divine spark within you." What a great way to greet a person! And what a fantastic way to try to view and perceive other people. In a world caught up with fashion and outward appearance, what a powerful perspective it is to try to see the spirit of another person rather than just his or her body or physical form.

The reason poetry is important to the physical and mental diets is that it causes us to have increased awareness, which lifts us to a higher realm of thought and places us above and in control of our appetites. But with the physical and mental, we are talking about the awareness of our senses, about what we can notice and be aware of through our sight, hearing, taste, smell, and touch.

> As we increase our spiritual perspective and awareness, we can literally lift ourselves out of the physical and view our body and our mind as tools that our spirit can use.

Spiritual awareness and perspective, on the other hand, go beyond this because they come from different sources and are far more insightful and transcending. As we increase our spiritual perspective and awareness, we can literally lift ourselves out of the physical and view our body and our mind as tools that our spirit can use. Physical appetites, in this context, are simply one part of our bodily tool, one aspect over which our spirit has control. The shape and weight and capacities of that physical tool are then at the command of the spirit.

Spiritual awareness and perspective is actually, in and of itself, a spiritual appetite, one of those marvelous, higher forms of appetite of which we can never have too much and for which we need no bridle or discipline. But it is an acquired appetite, one we have to cultivate and develop.

We need, first of all, to be convinced that seeing people (or things or situations) spiritually is more interesting and more enjoyable than seeing them physically. We have to believe that the attractiveness of a person's spirit is more important than the attractiveness of his or her body. We have to believe that we can learn something from everyone, and we have to really want to see our unfolding lives, and the lives of others, as the unfolding of God's plan rather than as mere chance or circumstance.

Earlier, we suggested that poetry could be used as a tool for increasing sensory awareness. Could it help with spiritual awareness? Certainly there is such a thing as spiritual poetry and poems about spiritual things, and trying to write that kind of poem could certainly enhance our spiritual awareness. Much of the Holy Bible is essentially poetry. The book of Isaiah is poetry; the Proverbs and the Psalms are poetry; much of the New Testament, particularly Christ's own words, as in the Sermon on the Mount, reads like poetry.

But whether you try to write spiritual poetry or not, you can think in a spiritually poetic way. Here are three challenges, each of which will increase and magnify your spiritual perspective and awareness. Think of them as "spiritual poetry."

1. *Take prayer notes.* Have a pad and a pen in your hands as you pray. Ask and listen. Pause and wait. Open your mind and your spirit to impressions and answers. Take notes on what you receive. Any impressions that come during earnest prayer constitute spiritual awareness.

2. *Keep an "ask journal."* When you ask God for something, write it down and keep track of it along with any nudges or impressions that come to you as you are asking for it. The impressions may alter or edit what you ask for. Look back over past entries often, and be aware of how the answers and the blessings are coming to you.

> It has been said that the difference between man and God can be stated in two words: *awareness* and *perspective.*
>
> He is aware of all and sees from every perspective.

3. *Ask for the quality of "Namaste."* Directly ask God to help you to see people's spirits and to be aware of their hearts. Ask to see their divine spark and to see them a little more as God sees them. Ask for this extra perception to apply also to how you see yourself.

It has been said that the difference between man and God can be stated in two words: *awareness* and *perspective.* He is aware of all and sees from every perspective. Enhancing our spiritual awareness and perspective is thus the greatest spiritual appetite and the most direct route to the ultimate goal of eternity: becoming, ever so gradually, more like our God.

CHAPTER 29

THE SPIRITUAL UN-BRIDLE

Compare to Chapters 9 and 19

Back in the physical and mental diet sections, we paid homage to James for the scriptural bridle metaphor. "We put bits in the horses' mouths," said James, an apostle of the New Testament, "that they may obey us; and we turn about their whole body." To become "perfect men," he said, we must be "able also to bridle" our bodies, our expressions, our appetites, and our tongues. In another scripture, a father gives his son this advice: "See that ye bridle all your passions, that ye may be filled with love."

As we emphasized earlier, one reason the horse is such a perfect metaphor is that horses are extraordinarily strong, remarkable, and beautiful creatures than can serve us in ways that are exciting and thrilling as well as useful. There is nothing quite like a horse at full gallop, especially if you are on its back, moving with it and feeling its grace and power. One of the great gifts of mortality is our physical and mental passions and appetites. When we bridle these horses, we fulfill our purposes and reach our potential.

However, the spiritual appetite is different from physical and mental appetites. It is only our spiritual appetites that serve and save us rather than snarl or snare us.

A HIGHER KIND OF CONTROL

There are two great and important ways to control and master our physical and mental appetites and make these gifts of mortality work for us rather than against us:

1. Bridle them and hold them in check, making them serve our will and give us joy rather than carrying us away.

2. Cultivate and develop our spiritual appetites to the point that they supersede our physical and mental appetites.

To reiterate yet again, our spiritual appetites need no bridle. They are a different kind of horse that we can totally trust and that will always take us home. With spiritual appetites (remember that spiritual appetites are for scripture, for prayer, for peace, for insight to the mind and will of God), there is no excess, no way to "gulp and guzzle." Rather, we "feast" and can never reach the point of too much. Obviously, we still need balance in our lives, but we can trust this horse to give us line upon line, to take us as far as we can go on any given day, to take us past, or over, or around, or through whatever dangers or challenges lie in our path.

OUR THREE HORSES

Remember that the physical and mental horses still live in our pasture, and we must ride them, too, always with a bridle and always in control so that they gradually become better and more manageable horses. Somehow, though, even as we love and enjoy and use the mental and physical horses, we long to spend more and more time riding bareback and without reins or bridle on the spiritual horse.

Over time, as we nurture and magnify the spiritual horse, we begin to learn how to become "horse whisperers" who can communicate constantly and with perfect understanding. Unlike the physical and mental horses, which we keep always under our watchful control, the spiritual horse has complete freedom, because we trust it even more than we trust ourselves. Thus it reveals things to us, drawing us toward its true master and giving us guidance as to how to handle the other two horses.

We learn that if we ride the spiritual horse first each morning and last each night, the other horses behave better during the day. We learn that whenever we are riding the spiritual horse, the other two follow along obediently, giving us no trouble whatsoever.

Sometimes we receive criticism for riding the spiritual horse. Some say we are extremists and that we are a little strange, like the horse we ride. They say that they are not even sure that what we are riding is a horse, because it looks different and acts different. Some make fun of the horse and of us when we are riding it.

We begin to notice that the spiritual horse really is different, and gradually we realize that it is actually not a horse at all but something different, something more magical—like Pegasus or like a unicorn! We tell others that and they scoff, assuring us that horses can't fly and that there is no such thing as a unicorn and that we are only imagining things. "Give up on this crazy idea," they tell us. "There are no unicorns, and if there were, you certainly couldn't ride it bareback, so come back to riding regular horses like the rest of us, and don't be so strict with the bridle. Let the regular horses have their head once in a while so you can live a little."

However, by now we know that the winged horse or the unicorn is real and that we can trust it and ride it, bridle-less, and that it will take us

> We learn that if we ride the spiritual horse first each morning and last each night, the other horses behave better during the day. We learn that whenever we are riding the spiritual horse, the other two follow along obediently, giving us no trouble whatsoever.

to the right destination and give us joy all along the way. We long to meet its master. We even get the idea that if we could take along the other two horses, with the master's help, they would one day be able to fly, too.

CHAPTER 30

REVIEW OF THE PRINCIPLES AND PRACTICES OF THE SPIRITUAL DIET

Compare to Chapters 10 and 20

As we review the basic principles and practices of the spiritual diet, it will be helpful to think back to the principles and practices of the physical and mental diets in Chapters 10 and 20. By glancing through them first, you will be able to see how similar and yet how different the spiritual diet is. You may also want to recommit yourself to the physical and mental diets if there are parts on which you have been slipping a bit.

On both the physical and the mental lists, the practices do not have to become tasks or things to check off or added burdens in our lives. Rather, they can simply become good habits—things we get used to doing and thus do naturally and easily.

As you review those principles and practices, notice how the physical and the mental match up. Physical food and our physical bodies and this physical earth truly are metaphors or "types" for all other appetites. Learning to control how we eat and how we enjoy the physical is the perfect school for learning how to use our minds and how to bridle all of our appetites (and make them work for our joy and our salvation rather than let them enable our destruction).

But the spiritual horse does not take the initiative like the physical and mental horses. It does not force or coerce us. It waits for us to call it and coax it, to use our agency and our gift of choice to make our own decision to mount up and ride.

The spiritual diet, however, is very different. As has been emphasized, it is about feasting rather than fasting and about trusting rather than bridling.

The physical and mental horses (appetites) of mortality, beautiful and empowering though they can be, will, if unbridled, carry us away from God and kill us both physically and spiritually. But the spiritual horse is of a different breed which, when trusted and honored, will always take us home. Our spiritual appetites are to know God, to serve God, to be more like God, to draw near to God, to love God, and to return to God.

But the spiritual horse does not take the initiative like the physical and mental horses. It does not force or coerce us. It waits for us to call it and coax it, to use our agency and our gift of choice to make our own decision to mount up and ride. Consequently, the principles and practices we must understand for the spiritual diet are rather different from those we've learned for the physical and mental diets.

Fifteen simple principles of the spiritual diet:

1. The earth, in all its variety, and everything in it—your body and all of this infinite-variety mortality—is a great gift from God.

2. Your body and your brain are godlike additions to your spirit, given here in mortality for the first time in eternity. And the spirit with the body forms the soul of man.

3. Still, the real you is and will always be the spiritual you, the eternal spiritual child of God, now given the added tools of a physical body and mind in order that you might experience more fully and gradually gain the awareness and perspective that makes you ever so slightly and ever so gradually more like God.

4. With these mortal gifts comes agency, which is the choice of whether we will use mortality or allow mortality to use us.

5. Your spirit has at its command and its disposal your body and your brain, which can become its extensions and tools if they are bridled or its destruction and demise if they are not.

6. Beyond that, the ultimate tool, which can extend your awareness eternally, is the spirit of God, which Christians would call the Holy Spirit.

7. Spiritual appetites are for prayer, scripture, service, inspiration, and the influence of the Spirit. They all lead us to want to be closer to and more like God. Spiritual appetites turn us outward as well as inward. They prompt empathy and service.

8. When they are cultivated and magnified, spiritual appetites supersede and exert control over mental and physical appetites. This "shift of horses" is even better than a bridle. Making that choice is the selection of God's will over our will, and it acknowledges that he, not you, is the captain of your soul.

9. The spiritual appetite is as different from the physical and mental appetites as the loaves and fishes of Jesus were different from ordinary food. It increases as it is consumed, and it gives us an

abundance mentality. Unlike physical things, our possession of spiritual things increases as we give them away.

10. Slowing down the physical and the mental can speed up the spiritual.

11. Our mortal challenge is to control and bridle the appetites of body and mind and to cultivate and magnify the appetites of the spirit.

12. The spirit, like the body, needs constant nourishment and hydration, and if we wait until we are extremely thirsty before drinking living water, we will experience, without really even being aware of it, chronic spiritual dehydration. Cultivated, encouraged, and prayed for, the thirst for living water can become more powerful than physical thirst.

13. Spiritual feasting is done by receiving the gifts of the Spirit as we feel and express gratitude. The expression of appreciation to God expands both our awareness and our joy.

14. As we learn to recognize and welcome spiritual appetites, we can feast on both the Word and the will of God.

15. The spiritual perspective is always beautiful and always poetic.

Seven simple practices of the spiritual diet (the habits of choosing the right half):

1. Each day, do not eat any physical food (e.g., toast or orange juice) or mental food (e.g., the newspaper or social media) until you have had some spiritual food (e.g., the scriptures and prayer).

2. Pray "evening, and morning, and at noon." Take prayer notes and keep an ask journal. Sip and savor the word and the communication of God. Opt consciously for God's will, and maintain that desire. Regularly, set aside a day to fast and to offer an extended prayer of thanksgiving and praise.

3. Cultivate inspiration by asking for and then acting on spiritual nudges or impressions each day.

4. Add some spiritual music that inspires you to your playlists.

5. Carry scripture with you. Consider carrying a different set of scriptures during each season.

6. Strive to see people's spirit rather than their body. (Ask for "Namaste.")

7. Use an hour of the Sabbath day to spiritually create the week ahead.

Different horse, different principles, different practices—but these are the ones that convert diet into discipleship!

DIET REDEFINED

Now, let me get personal again and set aside the horses-as-appetites metaphor for a moment (we will come back to it). Try for a moment to think of yourself as your eternal spirit, which currently inhabits a mortal form. Not a physical and mental being who occasionally has a spiritual experience but a spiritual being who is currently having a physical and mental experience on this mortal earth.

You, your spirit you, has a couple of fantastic tools at its disposal—your brain and your body. You (your spirit) can use your brain/body tool in so many ways. The mind has vastly more power and potential than we generally understand or use. You can program it to seek out and recognize whatever you want it to. You can use it in small ways (like an alarm clock that wakes you when you will it to) or in large

> You are not a physical and mental being who occasionally has a spiritual experience but a spiritual being who is currently having a physical and mental experience on this mortal earth.

ways (like programming it to warn you of danger or to wonder at beauty or to develop an embryonic idea within its subconscious). You can also program your body to be more responsive to stimulus or to ward off infection or to heighten or sharpen its senses.

Besides the powerful (and vastly underused) tools of brain and body, we also have access to ultimate power, awareness, and perspective because of our capacity to plug into the Holy Spirit—which is to Christians the third personage of the godhead. (Think of the brain as a powerful but limited laptop computer that can connect to the limitless mainframe and data cloud of the Spirit.) While we can't program the Holy Ghost, we can access its enormous power and perspective and hook up wirelessly to whatever insights and inspirations we truly need.

Think about that: The vastly powerful and underused tool of mind and brain, given, for the first time, during this mortality, is completely programmable by the real you (your eternal spirit). And the ultimate awareness, perspective, and illumination source and guidance system of the Holy Ghost is always available for connection.

There are three basic ways to approach a day. One is to get up and just see what happens to you, being totally passive and reactive. The second is to make a list, plan the day, and go out and try to check everything off, being always proactive and in control. On the surface, this second option sounds like the best choice—and it certainly is what most people either try to do or think they should be doing.

The third alternative is to get up and program and pray. Let me explain.

First, program your mind by essentially telling it that you want it to use its full capacity to give you awareness and perspective as the day unfolds. Instruct your brain to seek and find awareness of beauty, of taste, of people and their needs and feelings, of ideas and connections, of new ways to see and do things, and, most of all, of God's will and of what he wants you to see and think and give and do. Issue to your brain the programming command to sip and savor life and the good and important things in it. And program your mind to gather and discover the empathetic perspective of how things look to others, how seeming coincidences fit together, how opportunities could be developed and problems solved, and how God views things and responds to people.

Second, pray for the Spirit to take you beyond even the expanded capacities of your mind and to give to you additional awareness and perspective of all these things—and to give you the impressions, nudges, and guidance that will allow you to do what God wants you to do that day rather than what you want, what he knows is best rather than what you think is best.

You see, the second approach to a day (planning and being proactive) and the desire to force the day and its circumstances to go as we want leads to frustration and often to false paths, because it is based on the false premise that we control things and that we know what is best for us and those around us.

So when we try, day in and day out, to take that second approach, we end up finding ourselves "kicking against the pricks,"[40] as the scripture says, constantly trying to force things (and other people and situations and even time itself) to go the way we planned them. But things never quite go as planned or conform to what we had envisioned.

The real problem with this approach (beyond the frustration) is that we miss so much. Trying to use the brain to check off the things on our lists no matter what, rather than using its greater and more important capacity to give us added awareness and perspective, wastes the mind's capacity and puts it to a task for which it is less suited. Most importantly, by focusing on our own will, we lose sight of God's will.

When we take the program-and-pray alternative, we still have goals, we still may very well make a list, and we certainly still plan. The difference is that we do it prayerfully, trying to get as much guidance as we can in advance of the day. And we do it as a tentative, best-effort plan, admitting both to God and to ourselves that we know way too little to do a final plan and acknowledging that our desire is to do his will and not ours.

This attitude is the perfect preparation for programming the brain and then praying to the Spirit for all we can muster of awareness and perspective and for the added measure that the Spirit can bring. Then we move out into life, tentative plan in hand, with both our own limited brains and the unlimited Spirit working in tandem to reveal to us the beauties, the opportunities, and God's will for the moments that make up the day ahead.

We trust God's guidance, we expect it because we have asked for it, and we know that its ultimate source is connected to our soul. The day becomes an adventure and a serendipitous feast.

BACK TO THE THREE HORSES AND THE TWO BRIDLES

Programming the body and the brain, of course, is preparation for bridling the physical and mental horses. Mortal appetites, passions, and senses become trained to open us to greater awareness, perspective, beauty, and connections with others. We become beneficially connected to the horses and work with them even as we master and bridle them. They extend and enhance us and bring us joy. Praying for the guidance of the Spirit and for the impressions and nudges and guidance that give us God's gifts and lead us to his will is an advanced way of riding the winged horse and letting it take us home.

"Diet," in this context, means so much more than the conventional definition. It is the sequential training of two horses and the subsequent discovery of a third horse that is so much more, that lifts and trains us and takes us to a new home.

The marvelous bridling metaphor of James becomes the framework (and the key to understanding) three levels of truth: physical, mental/emotional, and spiritual. Appetites, passions, and desires transform from our obsessions and potential addictions into first our servants, then our friends, and finally our spiritual prompters and partners. Within this paradigm, life becomes joyous and daily living becomes more exciting, more positive, and more meaningful.

We have consistently given the New Testament James the credit for the horse-and-bridle metaphor around which this book centers, so let us end by expanding that symbolism (and the words of James) even further: The bit, like the tongue, is in the mouth, and the mouth is the place we have to have control over—both in terms of the words that come out of it and in terms of the food we put into it. The bit allows us to turn the powerful body of the horse, just as the tongue is the part of the body that we have to control if we wish not to hurt others or ourselves with our words.[41] Likewise, bridling what goes into the mouth allows us to turn our own bodies into the kind of bodies we want them to be and direct them toward the wellness we want to find.

Bridles, in actuality and in metaphor, are small things that control large things. They are devices that allow us to have control over things that, unbridled, are stronger than we are. Horses, in actuality and in metaphor as an appetite or passion, are large and very powerful things that must be bridled in order to be controlled.

Another scriptural prophet named Alma also used the bridle metaphor when he said, "See that ye bridle your passions, that ye may be filled with love." I think this is a marvelous phrase, first because it distinguishes between passion and love but even more because it teaches us that feelings, passions, and appetites grow purer and more beautiful when we learn to control and direct them and when we apply them correctly and point them in the directions God wants. We grow and expand our love not by letting our passions run away with us but by mastering them. We get the most joy out of a horse not by letting it run away with us but by bridling it.

Yesterday, an early spring day before I finished this book, I rode up a lovely canyon on a horse that took me much further and much faster than I could have gone on my own. I saw more, felt more, and loved more than

I could have without that horse, and it was the bridle that kept the joy from turning into danger.

The Half Diet is all about bridling and being filled with love. Appetite is not the enemy but a powerful asset and ally to be used and appreciated and *bridled.*

Appetite, when bridled, is a source of joy and love. A bridled horse becomes trained and soon starts to take us where we want to go almost automatically, with only a very light touch from the reins. A trained appetite can start to take us to the right foods in the right quantities almost automatically, without us having to constantly rein it in and hold it back.

> The Half Diet is all about bridling and being filled with love. Appetite is not the enemy but a powerful asset and ally to be used and appreciated and *bridled.*

The Half Diet is, essentially, about a bridle. As we discipline ourselves to eat half, our appetites gradually change from demanding quantity to demanding quality and begin to take us to where we want to be with very little pressure from our conscious reins. But the initial discipline and training is hard, and we need all the help we can get.

The most important thing about the whole bridling idea, as James and Alma make so clear, is that it works mentally and spiritually as well as physically. The things that the physical diet can do for your body have counterparts in the things that the mental diet can do for your brain and that the spiritual diet can do for your soul.

May you learn it all—for yourself.

ENDNOTES

1. Wootan, Margo. "Why It's Hard to Eat Well and Be Active in America Today." *Center for Science in the Public Interest*, 2014. http://www.cspinet.org/nutrition-policy/food_advertising.html

2. Abbey, Edward. *Desert Solitaire: A Season in the Wilderness*. New York: Ballantine Books, 1968.

3. Clash, James M. "Because It's There." *Forbes.com*, October 29, 2001. http://www.forbes.com/global/2001/1029/060.html

4. "Each One Matters." *Angelfire.com*. http://www.angelfire.com/ca4/angelwing1/each1matters.html

5. Conant, Eve. "Nap Quest."*Newsweek*, February 11, 2007. http://www.newsweek.com/nap-quest-104733

6. James 3:3 (King James Version).

7. James 3:2 (King James Version).

8. Alma 38:12 (*Book of Mormon*).

9. Hellmich, Nanci. "Study Suggests Eating Slowly Translates to Eating Less." *USA Today*, November 15, 2006. http://usatoday30.usatoday.com/news/health/2006-11-15-slower-eating_x.htm

10. Cummings, E. E. "55." *95 Poems*. New York: Harcourt Brace Jovanovich, 1958.

11. Honoré, Carl. *In Praise of Slow: How a Worldwide Movement Is Challenging the Cult of Speed*. Toronto: Vintage Canada, 2004. Pp. 4–5.

12. Ibid.

13. Honoré, Carl. *Under Pressure: Rescuing Children from the Culture of Hyper-Parenting*. Toronto: Knopf Canada, 2008. P. 162.

14. Honoré, Carl. *In Praise of Slow: How a Worldwide Movement Is Challenging the Cult of Speed*. Toronto: Vintage Canada, 2004. P. 247.

15. Luke 10:40 (King James Version).

16. Luke 10:41 (King James Version).

17. Luke 10:42 (Common English Bible).

18. Kipling, Rudyard. "If—." *Rewards and Fairies.* New York: Doubleday, 1910.

19. Moses 3:5 (*Pearl of Great Price*).

20. James 4:3 (King James Version).

21. Thoreau, Henry David. *Walden.* New York: Thomas Y. Crowell & Co., 1910.
    P. 430.

22. Newport, Frank. "More Than 9 in 10 Americans Continue to Believe in God."
    Gallup.com, June 3, 2011. http://www.gallup.com/poll/147887/americans-
    continue-believe-god.aspx.

23. Psalm 46:10 (King James Version).

24. Pratt, Parley P. *Key to the Science of Theology.* Liverpool: F. D. Richards, 1855.

25. Isaiah 40:31 (King James Version).

26. Mark 2:27 (New International Version).

27. Section 59 (*Doctrine and Covenants*).

28. Proverbs 3:8 (King James Version).

29. Ibid.

30. John 4:10 (King James Version).

31. John 4:14 (King James Version).

32. Ephesians 6:12 (King James Version).

33. 2 Peter 1:5 (Amplified Bible).

34. Helaman 3:35 (*Book of Mormon*).

35. Moroni 7:48 (*Book of Mormon*).

36. Psalm 55:17 (King James Version).

37. Alma 34:20 (*Book of Mormon*).

38. Lewis, C. S. *The Lion, the Witch and the Wardrobe.* London: Geoffrey Bles, 1950.

39. Philippians 2:12 (King James Version).

40. Acts 26:14 (King James Version).

41. James 3:3; 5–6 (King James Version).

ACKNOWLEDGMENTS

Thanks to our publisher, Christopher Robbins, and all the folks at Familius for caring about what readers care about, and to David Miles for design and to Brooke Jorden for layout and editing.

Thanks to Kathy Kidd and Darla Isackson for early editing, and to Lindsay Sandberg for later editing. Thanks most of all to the thousands of readers/dieters who initially read this book as a column-by-column series and who lost literally tons of weight and provided me with great feedback.

And thanks to Maurine and Scot Proctor who initially published much of the diet, in installments, within *Meridian*, their excellent online magazine.

MORE PRAISE FOR
THE HALF-DIET DIET

(These comments and endorsements came in from readers of the weekly article installments and the original book written under the pseudonym of Dr. Bridell.)

"All of your concepts just ring TRUE." —KS

"After looking at and trying nearly every diet out there, your whole program has made total sense to both my husband and me. I have lost twenty pounds with more to go, and he has lost fifty, not gained any back, and has more to go. Thank you very much for your timely and inspirational series. We're really looking forward to the book. I am looking forward to sharing it with our children!" —EE

"Your weekly articles have been such a great help to me. I have lost thirty-three pounds by putting into action all of your suggestions." —CM

"I have already enjoyed sharing the concepts and incorporating them. It has been a spiritual journey." —VH

"I have used the ideas and suggestions to help my friend lose sixty-eight pounds." —RH

"When I first started, 'eat half' was a challenge. After all, if I was eating a dozen chocolate chip cookies a day, then would I lose weight if I only ate six? But when I stopped snacking and truly cut down my portion sizes, the light bulb went on. I've lost thirty pounds." —TK

"I've been working and working for years to get this weight off that came on during years of infertility treatments, and with the Half Diet, it's finally working." —SA

"I absolutely swear by the eat-half diet, and I loved the spiritual advice, too." —KS

"The connection between the physical and the spiritual is the best part of the Half Diet plan!!" —PH

"The words and concepts and most of all the 'spirit' of the whole diet resonates with me . . . with my soul." —DM

"Your ideas are so different from the usual run-of-the-mill diet, as you use spiritual principles. I think this is the only way we can really achieve anything of value." —JG

"Your diet has given me thoughtful reflection on a lot of habits or attitudes I did not even know I had . . . [it] has made me more aware of choices in a lot of different areas." —KP

"As I read, your diet feels like revelation." —PW

"This has been a great journey for me. I have been amazed at the way that I have been taught the Gospel through this diet, which has addressed the spirit as well as the body." —LS

"This stuff is amazing!" —ER

"The half-plate idea (especially when eating out) has helped me control my portions. I try using a smaller plate at home and listening to what my body is saying." —JF

"What worked for me: eating half portions, slowly, with a glass of water beforehand. Being thankful, savoring the food, and relating what I can to the spiritual self as well. The idea is great." —BE

"I have seen a change in my physical body, but really the best change is in my spiritual body. Thank you, thank you. I have learned so much and been so motivated by this wonderful adventure." —KB

"Fun, down to earth, and easy to understand and implement." —CB

"Dr. Bridell, my husband lost thirty-six pounds in six weeks using your diet. When he went to see his doctor, he told him he needed to reweigh him because the nurse must not have gotten the weight right. He couldn't believe the scale was accurate and wanted to know how he was able to lose the weight. We gave the doctor your web address and I know of at least five people he has given it to. He says he will give it to all of his overweight patients. As for ourselves, everyone wants to know how my husband has lost all this weight. We have given this out to many people." —JG

"Thank you, Dr. Bridell, for your really different way of looking at weight maintenance. It's ahead of its time in melding the physical and spiritual." —DW

"Whenever I realize that I am in 'gulp and guzzle' mode, I stop and down-shift into 'sip and savor' mode. Tying your principles into the mental and spiritual elements of life make this diet easier to stick with." —SS

"It's common sense, and I like that it involves spiritual principles that will help me with the problems behind my overeating." —RB

"My friends and I are starting a support group based on the principles of the Half Diet." —KS

"I gave the Half-Diet Diet to my friend, and it was the beginning of a whole new person in her." —LW

"I am enthused with your ideas! And it only makes sense that our eating experiences would be multifaceted, since we are made up of body and spirit." —NS

"As a compulsive eater, I've found that using a twelve-step program in concert with your plan has blessed me very much. I have used your 'diet' as my food plan and to define my abstinence, and it has greatly blessed my life." —AP

"I have read a lot of diet and self-help books through the years, and yours is by far the very best. The advice is so simple yet so profound, and I love your writing style. It is very straightforward and to the point, not 'wordy,' as so many advice books are." —JR

"Simple comment: I love the way your diet works." —MM

"I was not really overweight, but as I blended principles from the 'eat half' diet into my personal eating habits, I gradually lost over ten pounds and have maintained my weight at a lower level." —MZ

"I love the new way I have of thinking about food and life. It is amazing how bridling even the passion for food helps me to be more aware and contemplative of the things around me." —HC

"I have noticed that you are right about my body (when intake is limited to half) craving good food to get the nutrition it needs. I have studied nutrition for years, and I know all about what not to eat, but learning what TO eat has been a challenge. This 'eat half' concept has really motivated me to dig into my huge healthy recipe collection and start learning how to feed myself and my family well." —JM

"The Half-Diet Diet has made a profound difference in our family. Your 'diet' is the most effective approach we have read; the results are gratifying, and the effort has been made so much easier as we understand and appreciate the correlation between mind, body, and spirit." —LM

"I am an avid fan. Thank you for your approach and insight; it works for me. It is the best approach I've seen so far." —JB

"Your column has given me a different kind of hope and a renewed desire to truly lose weight for all of the right reasons." —SN

"I must be ready to hear your counsel because the correlation between spiritual and physical is becoming more evident to me. I feel more spiritually blessed when I have the grace to restrain my physical appetites." —KM

"I haven't lost a lot of weight (ten pounds), but I have changed how I look at a diet. I love the 'eat half' way of eating. I've been trying to eat more sensibly for years. This has helped me look at life a different way. I love the metaphor of the horse and bridle." —BB

"The combination of physical and mental is so important, and you have combined the two wonderfully. I'm trying to convince my wife to try it." —DH

"I feel better! I look better!" —KK

"It has given 'diet' a whole different meaning." —MS

"As a doctor and an amateur theologian, I would like to observe that the Half-Diet Diet has an approach that seems to be an 'East meets West meets Gospel' approach to well-being." —CC

"I am so very grateful that a diet book that looks at the spiritual side has finally come to my attention. I believe that the having a good and righteous spirit is the very best foundation for success in everything. I did find that reducing portions helped me to lose quite a bit of weight already . . . forty pounds." —HK

"The Lord has blessed (and cursed) me with strong appetites and emotions. He has also personally admonished me to control (or bridle) them. I know that as I am able to accomplish this task, I will be able to emphasize the positive aspects of such a gift and do great things. Your diet has most certainly been an essential tool in this pursuit." —JB

"I have faithfully read this new and revolutionary diet, trying to digest as much of it as I can. I have loved every morsel." —KL

"I love it and look forward to having it to share with a very dear friend of mine so that we can work the program together." —GH

"I am interested in a healthy lifestyle, and although I do not struggle with weight problems, I have family members and friends who do. Your sensible principals just sound right, not only for people who have weight to lose but those of us who just want to feel better." —CB

"I believe in the principles and have applied them successfully. It is the epitome of sage and sane advice." —JF

"Thank you for putting into words what I've felt and thought about for the past several years." —JW

"I have lost fifteen pounds so far and am continuing to use it in my life. Thank you for bringing new ways of looking at things to me." —MB

"Thanks for your delightful and practical writing. It has been a long time since I have bridled a horse, but I find this new kind of bridle challenging and delightful." —EC

"Great approach! I've made wonderful changes in my thinking and my eating." —TW

"I have discovered flavors and tastes I never knew of before. Somehow I feel so much more at peace and in tune with the Spirit." —WT

"I will be telling family and friends about your diet—anyone who wants to lose weight and, especially, anyone who feels the need for more spiritual enlightenment (that describes most all of us)." —SD

"Much more reasonable and doable than all the other fad diets out there. I think your approach is the best way to achieve a PERMANENT healthy lifestyle and the best way to respect the gift of our bodies." —GD

"We have decided to start an enrichment health class using your chapters as text and adding exercise ideas and group support to help us all with the life changes essential to lose weight and reach optimum health." —AB

"I have long believed in the true principles you teach . . . that our physical fitness is so closely connected to our emotional and spiritual fitness." —SR

"The Half-Diet Diet has had such profound effect. It helps us bridle our passions and gain more joy in physical and spiritual ways." —LN

"My weight loss now exceeds twenty pounds, and my colleagues cannot believe that my lifestyle adjustment is working." —SA

"I've been in conflict with eating disorders most of my life. I'm hopeful this will be my spiritual, mental, and physical breakthrough." —KB

"I completely agree that solving a weight-gain problem can only be successfully accomplished by addressing the spiritual roots of the problem." —CR

"Thank you for helping me realize just what I am doing to myself. I am bound and determined to stick with this and be a better me, in all aspects of my life. I think I understand better just what our bodies can do and should be like." —DP

"I love the balance between physical and spiritual, especially the section on fasting." —EB

"Thanks so much for your insight. Please continue to minister to those with a heartbreaking addiction that is just as destructive as drugs or alcohol but doesn't receive the same help or compassion that other addictions have." —DG

"I lost my wife two years ago after thirty-six years of marriage and five children. My adjustment has been difficult and I have looked for things to keep me from gaining weight and doing other unhealthy things. Your articles have given me many good, practical ideas." —JF

"A diet book like this, that discusses more than just food, is one I would very much like to read and share." —CB

"The Half Diet plan is simple. Simple to start and actually not that hard to keep going, either. It just makes sense." —JS

"What you are saying does make things clear to me. I especially like the way it ties the physical, mental, and spiritual together and how the same basic principles can be applied to all three. I know in my case that when I apply correct principles to the physical and mental aspects of my being, the spiritual aspect does much better." —KJ

"I have tried diet after diet after diet and have given up due to the failure that I felt. After reading and scanning the Half Diet, I feel like there is hope!" —CW

"What a diet! I have been 'enlightened' in more ways than one." —AR

"This poetic diet has slowed down my life as well as decreas[ed] my caloric intake." —KB

"Thank you for this wonderful diet. I am losing my weight slowly and so pleasantly!" —GC

"As I have read each installment, the principles espoused have all rung true with me. Some of the principles I had stumbled upon myself before I had read your diet, and you gave them a voice." —LH

"I haven't found words to express my gratitude for such an enlightening bunch of information. The food diet has helped me lose twenty pounds, but even that is not so valuable as the spiritual aspect of the diet." —AH

"One that has touched me is the principle of the living waters. Whenever I drink a glass of water, I think of the words 'living waters.' I love this comparison. I immediately think to myself, *Have I filled myself with living waters of the scriptures and the words of God as much as I craved the waters that fill my body many times a day?* I love the visual idea of the bridle." —LJ

"I especially have liked realizing how all the different pieces of the diet fit together. Understanding the mental and spiritual part of the plan has given me a much better understanding of how to handle the physical. I had just been diagnosed with type 2 diabetes when the book started appearing. Thus the diet has been, for me, a 'tender mercy.'" —MS

"My favorite part about your approach is the linking of the physical with the spiritual and mental/emotional. I don't believe any real, long-lasting benefits can happen without addressing all three." —TC

"I do appreciate so much the spiritual aspect, because I do believe that 'dieting' and eating issues are definitely more than just having 'will-power.'" —JR

"Thank you for a great new approach to dieting and life. I have a long way to go, but you've given me a way to go, and in 'bite-sized' pieces that really work." —LS

"The emotional and spiritual aspect of your series had a tremendous impact on my outlook so very often." —DF

"Thanks for the new perspective on life." —NR

"So much of what we need is just plain common sense, but we forget it. Thanks for putting it together so well. I particularly enjoy the spiritual aspect." —SH

"I have lost twelve pounds so far. I have to say that this is the first diet that's really made any sense to me, and I've realized that this is the first diet I haven't had anything to rebel against!! I have enjoyed eating all of my favorite foods, but I have also learned to gauge when I am reasonably filled. This is a new feeling, but I am learning to trust it, and it is working. And you were right . . . I am starting to crave more fruits and vegetables. It's also pretty amazing to think I have poetry inside of me." —CP

"Your diet is easy to follow and doesn't require special equipment, hassle, or frustration!" —RS

"This diet has totally changed the way I think about eating." —RP

"I love the horse analogies and how they helped me really understand the body/mind/spirit differentiation analogies." —SC

"Thanks for taking the time to address the entire realm of dieting and bringing to light one of our missions here on earth, which is to learn not only to control our appetites but also to understand, care for, and master our mortal bodies." —DA

"Excellent advice and help with physical as well as spiritual appetites." —MS

"I enjoy my food more even while I eat less (the quality of the food I eat has vastly improved as well as the kind of food I WANT to eat)!" —AT

ABOUT THE AUTHOR

RICHARD EYRE is a *New York Times* #1 bestselling author whose writing career has spanned four decades and whose books have sold in the millions. He has appeared on virtually all major national talk shows, including *Oprah* and *Today*, and has seen his books translated into a dozen languages. Together with his wife, Linda, he writes a syndicated weekly newspaper column and tries to keep up with their twenty-seven grandchildren. The Eyres currently spend most of their time traveling and speaking to audiences throughout the world about wellness, families, parenting, and life-balance. Richard and Linda live in Park City, Utah.

ABOUT FAMILIUS

Welcome to a place where parents are celebrated, not compared. Where heart is at the center of our families, and family at the center of our homes. Where boo-boos are still kissed, cake beaters are still licked, and mistakes are still okay. Welcome to a place where books—and family—are beautiful. Familius: a book publisher dedicated to helping families be happy.

VISIT OUR WEBSITE: www.familius.com

Our website is a different kind of place. Get inspired, read articles, discover books, watch videos, connect with our family experts, download books and apps and audiobooks, and along the way, discover how values and happy family life go together.

JOIN OUR FAMILY

There are lots of ways to connect with us! Subscribe to our newsletters at www.familius.com to receive uplifting daily inspiration, essays from our Pater Familius, a free ebook every month, and the first word on special discounts and Familius news.

BECOME AN EXPERT

Familius authors and other established writers interested in helping families be happy are invited to join our family and contribute online content. If you have something important to say on the family, join our expert community by applying at:

www.familius.com/apply-to-become-a-familius-expert

The most important work

you ever do will be within

the walls of your own home.